Claudia J. Carson
Anna S. Fritz
Elizabeth Lewis
John H. Ramey
David T. Sugiuchi
Editors

Growth and Development Through Group Work

Pre-publication
REVIEWS,
COMMENTARIES,
EVALUATIONS . . .

"This book is an antidote to the social toxicities that threaten to crush social work practice. It reawakens the reader to the dual role of social work with groups of addressing individual needs and social reform.

The recognition that something is amiss in social work practice constitutes a core challenge that this book addresses by pointing readers to the neglected connection that is social work's birthright: the relationship between private troubles and public issues."

Andrew Malekoff, MSW
Associate Executive Director,
North Shore Child and Family
Guidance Center,
Roslyn Heights, New York;
Editor, *Social Work with Groups*

"This well-written collection provides insights valuable to practitioners, educators, and researchers. Beginning with historical underpinnings, the chapters illustrate group work's many uses, enhancing readers' understanding of the group's value as a force for growth and development.

A unique section of the book titled 'Group Workers Facing New and Unpredictable Situations' provides stimulating examples of workers reaching out to unexplored areas of social need and expressing their feelings in the context of work in international, cross-cultural, and medical settings."

Paul Abels, PhD
Professor Emeritus,
California State University,
Long Beach, Department
of Social Work; President,
Association for the Advancement
of Social Work with Groups

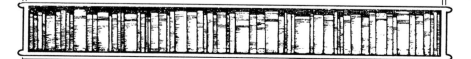

More pre-publication
REVIEWS, COMMENTARIES, EVALUATIONS . . .

"The chapters of this text consist of papers presented at the annual social group work conference that occurred exactly one month after September 11th, 2001. Similar to many conferences that took place shortly after that horrifying time, the participants were in various states of shock, and the conference became a forum to sort out what was occurring in the world.

Now, in 2004, this book can be seen as a snapshot of the thinking that occurred at this conference. A prominent theme throughout the book is the interconnectedness of private troubles and public issues. From describing group work's history and new areas of practice to providing practical teaching methods and techniques; from synthesizing new knowledge from research areas to an excellent summary of Ruby Pernell's legacy—each chapter found its footing in the deceptively simple idea that individuals cannot be seen as separate from the world without seriously distorting the individual and our world.

Group work's basic tenets of shared identity and mutual aid—what happens to one group member happens to us all—could not stand as more poignant exemplars for our post-9/11 world."

Aaron M. Brower, PhD
Professor, School of Soicial Work,
University of Wisconsin–Madison

"Following the tragedy and trauma of September 11th, 2001, the twenty-third annual Symposium on Social Work with Groups was held in Akron, Ohio. Participants traveled from all over the world to learn from and support one another. The conference's excellent proceedings, *Growth and Development Through Group Work,* fully captures and reaffirms group work's historic commitment to the creative integration of theory, practice, and research as well as its boundless spirit and proactive resilience.

Readers will be informed of group work history and its relevance for contemporary practice; important practice themes such as the organizational context of group work practice, the movement from group themes to broader social influence, group conflict, language barriers, and educational groups; group work education in the class and field; and of the contributions of research to group work practice."

Alex Gitterman, EdD
Professor of Social Work,
University of Connecticut
School of Social Work;
Co-editor, *The Legacy of William Schwartz: Group Practice As Shared Interaction*

The Haworth Press®
New York • London • Oxford

Growth and Development Through Group Work

THE HAWORTH PRESS
Titles of Related Interest

Group Work: Strategies for Strengthening Resiliency edited by Timothy D. Kelly, Toby Berman-Rossi, and Susanne E. Palombo

Social Work with Groups: Mining the Gold edited by Sue Henry, Jean East, and Cathryne Schmitz

Stories Celebrating Group Work: It's Not Always Easy to Sit on Your Mouth edited by Roselle Kurland and Andrew Malekoff

Crossing Boundaries and Developing Alliances Through Group Work edited by Jocelyn Lindsay, Daniel Turcotte, and Estelle Hopmeyer

Social Work with Groups: Social Justice Through Personal, Community, and Societal Change edited by Nancy E. Sullivan, Ellen Sue Mesbur, Norma C. Lang, Deborah Goodman, and Lynne Mitchell

The Mutual-Aid Approach to Working with Groups: Helping People Help One Another, Second Edition by Dominique Moyse Steinberg

Growth and Development Through Group Work

Claudia J. Carson
Anna S. Fritz
Elizabeth Lewis
John H. Ramey
David T. Sugiuchi
Editors

The Haworth Press®
New York • London • Oxford

The Haworth Press, Inc., 10 Alice Street, Binghamton, NY 13904-1580.

PUBLISHER'S NOTE
Identities and circumstances of individuals discussed in this book have been changed to protect confidentiality.

Cover design by Jennifer M. Gaska.

Library of Congress Cataloging-in-Publication Data

Symposium on Social Work with Groups (23rd : 2001 : Akron, Ohio, and Cleveland, Ohio)
    Growth and development through group work / Claudia J. Carson . . . [et al.], editors.
        p. cm.
    Includes bibliographical references and index.
    Papers from the Twenty-Third Annual Symposium on Social Work with Groups, held in Akron/Cleveland, Ohio, Oct. 11, 2001.
        ISBN 0-7890-2639-2 (hard : alk. paper) — ISBN 0-7890-2640-6 (soft : alk. paper)
        1. Social group work—Congresses. I. Carson, Claudia J. II. Title.
HV45.S955 2001
361.4—dc22
                                                                                        2004015419

This symposium is dedicated to the memory of Ruby Beatrice Pernell, who was among the earliest developers of the Association for the Advancement of Social Work with Groups (AASWG). In the United States, Canada, and many other places throughout the world, she taught, spoke, consulted, and wrote in favor of advancing the practice of social group work beyond neighborhood-centered work. On the international scene, she was one of several sage leaders chosen after World War II to help orient German culture to the more participatory democratic society of the United States. The long-term effects of those efforts show up in current history. Ruby worked on various aspects of the symposium right up to the day before her death in February 2001. We are deeply indebted to her for her devotion to group work and to AASWG, and in her memory, we lovingly dedicate this volume to her and commend its contents to present and future group workers to carry on her legacy.

CONTENTS

PART I: HISTORICAL PERSPECTIVES

PART II: CONTEMPORARY APPLIED GROUP WORK

PART III: EVOLVING GROUP WORK EDUCATIONAL APPROACHES

PART IV: GROUP WORKERS FACING NEW AND UNPREDICTABLE SITUATIONS

ABOUT THE EDITORS

Claudia J. Carson, MSSA, is Field Coordinator in the School of Social Work at Cleveland State University in Ohio. She is co-chair of the Northeast Ohio Chapter of the Association for the Advancement of Social Work with Groups, Inc. (AASWG), and co-chaired the Twenty-Third Annual International Symposium on Social Work with Groups in 2001.

Anna S. Fritz, MSSA, is a former faculty member of the Mandel School of Applied Social Sciences at Case Western Reserve University in Cleveland, Ohio. She is actively involved with the Northeast Ohio AASWG board.

Elizabeth Lewis, MSSA, is Professor Emeritus in the School of Social Work at Cleveland State University. She is co-founder and an active member of the Northeast Ohio Chapter of AASWG board, and is a member of the National Academies of Practice in Social Work.

John H. Ramey, MA in Soc. Adm., is Associate Professor Emeritus of Social Work at the University of Akron in Ohio. He has been active in the leadership of the AASWG since its inception and served as its General Secretary for more than 15 years. He has served as Editor of the *Social Work with Groups Newsletter* since 1985.

David T. Sugiuchi, MSSA, retired after four decades of social work practice with individuals, groups, and families. He is active in the National Association of Social Workers (NASW) and AASWG. He co-chaired the Twenty-Third Annual International Symposium on Social Work with Groups in 2001.

CONTRIBUTORS

Edith M. Anderson, MSW, is Assistant Field Coordinator and MSW Faculty Member at Cleveland State University. Prior to joining the faculty, she worked in direct practice where she facilitated treatment and task groups. As Director of Staff Development and Training in the Juvenile Justice System she worked at local, state, and national levels. Edith has worked with groups at the Young Women's Christian Association, American Management Association, and Services to Young Families.

Janice L. Andrews is Professor, University of Saint Thomas/College of Saint Catherine School of Social Work, where she chairs the policy content area and teaches social work history, progressive social work practice, and group work, and chairs student clinical research papers. She is a member of the board of AASWG and is Chair of the 2005 AASWG conference in Minneapolis. She publishes in a variety of journals and has given presentations in the United States, Canada, England, Norway, and Germany. She is co-author of the book *The Road Not Taken: A History of Radical Social Work in the United States* and is completing a book on the life and legacy of Gisela Konopka.

Toby Berman-Rossi, DSW, is Professor of Social Work, Barry University School of Social Work, where she teaches group work in the master's and doctoral programs. Prior to her work as a full-time educator, she worked with girls in adolescent inpatient psychiatry and with older persons in long-term care. Her twenty years of practice with groups prior to her teaching have enriched her classrooms. She has offered many presentations at professional conferences and symposia; has published in various journals, primarily on group work and practice with older persons; and has edited *Social Work: The Collected Writings of William Schwartz.* She is a member of the board of AASWG and is Immediate Past President of the Association.

Doug Beumer, LGSW, is a school social worker for Minneapolis public schools. His interests include family support, community building, international social work, and group work.

Catherine Coulthard, MSW, is a social worker with the Inflammatory Bowel Disease Program at Mount Sinai Hospital in Toronto, Canada. Her interests include involvement with peer-led support groups, direct clinical practice, and research.

Kathleen Holtz Deal, DSW, is Assistant Professor at the University of Maryland, School of Social Work, Baltimore, Maryland. She was a field instructor and leader of community mental health groups for many years. She currently teaches MSW practice courses and does research on student and field instructor development.

Mary Beth Gustafson, LGSW, is Intergenerational Coordinator for Minneapolis Public Schools and Service Coordinator in the Block Nurse Program at Southeast Seniors. She is interested in work with the geriatric population in the community setting.

Diane C. Haslett has worked with groups for over thirty years. Echoing the work begun by Rachelle Yarros in the early years of Hull House, in the 1980s she developed and implemented group work programs at Jane Addams Center—Hull House, including a drop-in center for young teens, sex education classes in conjunction with the Chicago Public Schools, and Lifelines, a multiservice center for teen parents. Currently she is Associate Professor and BASW Program Coordinator at the University of Maine, School of Social Work, Orono, Maine.

Lonnie R. Helton, PhD, is Associate Professor of Social Work at Cleveland State University, where he has been a faculty member for eleven years. Prior to joining academia, he worked for seventeen years as a social worker in the fields of mental health, health care, and developmental disabilities. He has co-authored two books and written extensively in the areas of multicultural practice, Appalachian studies, family intervention, and practice with children. He has developed and led groups in both inpatient and outpatient settings, serving children and families.

Stacy Husebo is Assistant Director and Clinical Social Worker at Face to Face Health and Counseling Services/Safe Zone, working with homeless and at-risk youth in St. Paul, Minnesota. She is committed to social activism and group work with youth.

Jürgen Kalcher was Professor at the Hamburg University of Applied Sciences, School of Social Work, from 1970 through 2000. His approach to social work has been widely influenced by social psychology. Now retired, he is still teaching in the field of social work with groups. He is also engaged in the advancement and development of social group work in Hamburg, Germany.

Timothy B. Kelly, PhD, is a Senior Research Fellow in Gerontological Practice at the School of Nursing, Midwifery and Community Health, Glasgow Caledonian University. Previously he was an Associate Professor of Social Work at Barry University in Miami Shores, Florida, where he taught group work. His practice experience includes serving as a social worker in a geriatric hospital, directing a day treatment program for older people living with a mental illness, and working in mental health centers. He has published articles in *Social Work with Groups, Social Work in Education,* and the *Journal of Social Work Education.* He currently is Secretary of AASWG.

Paule McNicoll is Associate Professor at the School of Social Work and Family Studies of the University of British Columbia, Vancouver, Canada, where she teaches group work at the BSW and MSW levels. She is a graduate of l'Université Laval (BA and BSW), the University of British Columbia (MSW), and the University of Washington (PhD). She is committed to the revitalization of group work, especially the use of the method for social justice purposes.

Patricia M. Merle, MSW, PhD, is co-founder and Director of Step by Step of Rochester, Inc., working with women who are or have been incarcerated. Using the strengths-based perspective as the foundation, Step by Step offers several eight-week structured workshops at correctional facilities, as well as weekend retreats, support groups, special events for women and their families, mentoring teams to help women in the transition process from prison, and programs for families of the incarcerated.

Helen Northen, PhD, is Distinguished Professor Emerita at the University of Southern California, where she taught social work practice and research for thirty years and was Director of the doctoral program. She is the author or co-author of numerous articles and several books, including *Clinical Social Work, Social Work with Groups,* and *Theories of Social Work with Groups.*

Brenda O'Connor, RN, BScN, is Research Coordinator in the Department of General Surgery at Mount Sinai Hospital in Toronto, Canada. Her interests include involvement with clinical trials in the Inflammatory Bowel Disease Program and with patient education and support.

Sarah Ann Schuh, LGSW, is a social worker with Davita, a company that provides outpatient kidney dialysis. Her interests include grief, loss, and hope; clinical social work; and group work.

Nancy Sullivan, PhD, RSW, is Associate Professor in the School of Social Work at Memorial University of Newfoundland, Canada. She is a longtime AASWG member and symposium participant and is Immediate Past Vice President of the Association.

Joanne Sulman, MSW, is Research Coordinator in the Department of Social Work at Mount Sinai Hospital in Toronto, Canada. Her research interests include the effectiveness of social group work practice in hospital settings.

At-Large Members:
Paul A. Abels, Costa Mesa, California
Janice L. Andrews, Minneapolis, Minnesota
Elisa Valladares Goldberg, New York, New York
Ella Lee Harris, Brooklyn, New York
Diane C. Haslett, Bangor, Maine
Flavio Francisco Marsiglia, Tempe, Arizona
Paule McNicoll, Vancouver, British Columbia, Canada
Denise Nerette, Miami, Florida
Robert M. Ortega, Ann Arbor, Michigan
Mary Wilson, Tivoli, Cork, Ireland

Chapter Representatives:
Southern California—Joan K. Parry, Vista, California
Connecticut—Susan Lalone, Danvers, Massachusetts
Florida—Susanne E. Palombo, Virginia Beach, Virginia
Georgia—Barry A. Burns, Snellville, Georgia
Germany—Ingrun Masanek, Norden, Germany
Illinois—Sally J. Mason, Chesterton, Indiana
Kentucky—Alison H. Johnson, Louisville, Kentucky
Long Island—Loretta Hartley-Bangs, Lindenhurst, New York
Massachusetts—Mary V. Lisbon, Jamaica Plain, Massachusetts
Michigan—Charles D. Garvin, Ann Arbor, Michigan
Minnesota—Rodney J. Dewberry, Minneapolis, Minnesota
New York Red Apple—Michael W. Wagner, Tappan, New York
Northeast Ohio—Ellen M. O'Leary, Youngstown, Ohio
Toronto—Barbara L. Muskat, Toronto, Ontario, Canada

Preface

In the fall of 2001, the Northeast Ohio Chapter of AASWG welcomed the Twenty-Third Annual Symposium on Social Work with Groups. Reaching this point had taken us on an extraordinary journey. We experienced significant losses as a group, both with the death of Ruby Pernell and also the illness of our co-chair, Dave Sugiuchi.

There were, of course, the normal bumps along the planning path, but finally we thought we were over the biggest hurdles and ready to move full speed and full vigor into the last phase of our journey. Little did we or the rest of the world know what lay ahead on September 11. The immediate aftermath of that horrific day led to a discussion of canceling or rescheduling the symposium. As you know, that was not the decision reached, and, in retrospect, was not the decision needed at that time.

Those who attended came with a sense of disbelief, but also a need to share their own experiences, reflect on what had occurred, and offer support to one another. The sense of "groupness" was extraordinary. As we shared our thoughts, feelings, ideas, and knowledge, we inevitably moved to the urgency of what we must all be about in the future development of group work.

From the Opening Plenary and the vitality of the Akron Steel Drum Band to the closing futuristic Breakfast Plenary, there continued to be an element of hope. Much of the hopefulness was building on the power of group work, especially in the present time of crisis, but also in continuing to build the future. How ironic it was that we found ourselves at the location of the "birthplace" of group work at a time when there was such a deep need to view the future through new lenses.

The following introduction provides a brief synopsis of the selected papers and plenaries. We are pleased to share them with you and hope that they will be utilized to strengthen the development of group work for future generations.

Claudia Carson, MSSA
Co-Chair, Twenty-Third Annual Symposium

Acknowledgments

The following people helped to plan and manage the Twenty-Third Annual Symposium of the Association for the Advancement of Social Work with Groups: Becky Adler, Pam Bradford, Molly Brudnick, Claudia Carson, Judy Fant, Ray Fant, Virginia Fitch, Anna Fritz, Paula Horton, Maggie Jackson, Elizabeth Lewis, Gail Long, Yvonne Matus, Pat Mitchell, Nellie O'Leary, John Ramey, Lynne Rose, Cazzell Smith, Gerald Strom, Dave Sugiuchi, Jay Toth, Tanya Vanderveen, and the late Ruby Pernell.

Two graduate assistants deserve recognition for their assistance prior to, during, and after the symposium: Special thanks to Katie Kessler and Jacqueline Minyard.

Our thanks also to the three cosponsoring universities: Case Western Reserve University, Cleveland State University, and the University of Akron. An additional thank-you goes to the Northeast Ohio Chapter of the AASWG.

Finally, a very special thank-you to the George Gund Foundation for their generous support.

Introduction

Claudia J. Carson
Anna S. Fritz
Elizabeth Lewis
John H. Ramey
David T. Sugiuchi

The Twenty-Third Annual Symposium on Social Work with Groups—
1923-2001 and Beyond: Growth and Development Through Group
Work—came together in Akron/Cleveland on October 11, 2001, at a
time when "beyond" seemed a large unknown. In the aftermath of
September 11, just one month earlier, when terrorist attacks in New
York City and Washington, DC, resulted in unspeakable losses for the
United States and elsewhere, there was a shared sense among symposium participants from around the country and around the world that
such events on U.S. soil have an unreality to them—an aura of disbelief. We needed desperately to affirm and experience together the underlying theme of the continuity of our work and its development,
which emerged as the symposium proceeded. Several presenters focused on group work roots and fundamental beliefs that carried us beyond the "disaster" stage of the national trauma we were experiencing, toward envisioning the group work of the future.

HISTORICAL PERSPECTIVES

Janice L. Andrews, in the opening plenary session, "The Legacy of
Ruby Pernell and Social Group Work" (Chapter 1), captured in brief
the efficacy of the group work method to teach human beings to survive, even embrace, differences of many kinds to form workable relationships. Pernell worked quietly and persistently at all levels of
human exchange to improve the human condition. Today, most poi-

gnantly, we need to have faith that our social group work skills and knowledge, applied locally, nationally, and internationally, are basic to the maintenance of our democratic society.

Presentations focused on group work theory and practice historically, informing contemporary group work and forcing attention to essential future directions, notably "Contributions of Research to Group Work" (Chapter 2) by Helen Northen, who urges social workers to evaluate, research, and present their findings about practice with groups. Prior to formal education for group work, leaders in group work agencies sought relevant knowledge about groups from other disciplines and from social casework. Northen provides the basis for the development of the scientific knowledge base for group work by examining its early educational beginnings. Examples are offered of research on group work that has contributed to successful outcomes for members. Northen's chapter is a call to professionals to reflect on and analyze their experience and research, for the purpose of continuing the development of scientific knowledge about social work with groups.

An invitational paper presented by Diane C. Haslett, "Group Work at Hull House: Lessons from the Past, Signposts for the Future" (Chapter 3), highlights Rachelle Yarros, a physician who lived and worked at Hull House during the late 1800s and early 1900s. Yarros's work is reviewed, addressing educational groups, research, and evaluation in the fields of sex education, contraception, and reproductive freedom. Haslett's chapter calls for today's group workers to reflect on their current practice, and how they might move from group worker to social change agent.

"Social Group Work in Germany: An American Import and Its Historical Development" (Chapter 4) by Jürgen Kalcher is a moving personal account that reflects on the concept of reeducating a whole people, developed at about 1943. Both British and American politicians and the military set out to change the norms of German society and, thereby, the Germans themselves. The focus is on a historical overview of an interdependent approach in Germany through the efforts of exiled German professionals in the United States and "daring American humanists," mostly social workers, who were able to shape successfully and convincingly a new democratic generation in Germany. The vehicle was social work with groups—an American import. Social group work as a method for democratizing and reeducating the Germans was brought to Germany by the "peace bringers," including some of our well-known group work pioneers who were successful because they were connected with real personal engagement.

CONTEMPORARY APPLIED GROUP WORK

Two authors conceptualize aspects of group work practice and teaching with focused clarity and direction applicable to current reality in group work. In "Conflict As an Expression of Difference: A Desirable Group Dynamic in Anti-Oppression Social Work Practice" (Chapter 5), Nancy Sullivan views conflict as a positive and functional force in the group process. Sullivan reflects on a time when social group work built on the "normal" socialization process and thus equipped group members with social competencies for effective and harmonious living, suggesting instead that we view conflict as "an expression of difference." By providing ten principles for desirable conflict in social group work and illustrating their use through vignettes, Sullivan invites practitioners to link the early purposes of social group work to their practice today.

In an invitational paper, "Putting Social Justice on the Agenda: Addressing Habitual and Social Barriers" (Chapter 6), Paule McNicoll examines the current organization of social work practice as it negatively effects the creation of groups that pursue social justice. By using an extended medical model, social work agencies have individualized social problems and separated them from elements of solution. To move toward a new vision of social work that would favor the creation of groups to pursue social justice, three particular barriers are identified. McNicoll also identifies some developments in the direction of the vision of social justice and moves on to begin to develop this vision based on a health promotion model for social work.

EVOLVING GROUP WORK EDUCATIONAL APPROACHES

Toby Berman-Rossi and Timothy B. Kelly illustrate ways in which we can help students integrate the dichotomy of private troubles and public issues into their practice approaches in "Using Groups to Teach the Connection Between Private Troubles and Public Issues" (Chapter 7). In an integrated generalist model of education and practice, this teaching should be infused throughout the curriculum. Berman-Rossi and Kelly demonstrate how the teaching of group work is the ideal content to help students see and use these connections and provide teaching tools and strategies to make explicit in class the practice skills for working with private troubles and public issues in groups. Their chapter addresses several areas, each with distinctive challenges for teaching and learning and requiring different strategies for the students, the profession, group work itself, and the agency setting on the subject matter of using groups. Sections focus on contexts, beginnings (contracting, group planning, assessment), middles or work phases (problem domains), and endings. Berman-Rossi and Kelly conclude by asking, "Who better to do this than group work?" This a most inspiring and useful presentation of core issues in group work education and practice—the simultaneous focus on private troubles and public issues.

"Restorative Education: Group-Centered Dialogue Between Students and Faculty at a Graduate School of Social Work" (Chapter 8) is the work of Stacey Husebo, Sarah Ann Schuh, Mary Beth Gustafson, and Doug Beumer. These recent social work graduates document a one-time forum between students and faculty to explore and experience collaborative teaching and learning in a school of social work. It is a microcosm of issues between participants with differing power resources and parallels the tasks between group members and social group workers. This radical approach to social group work education is practiced at a few selected schools of social work. This successful teaching/learning experience, developed by second-year social group work students at a Midwestern university, is promoted as an exciting and effective method for developing the social group work practitioner.

"Group Simulation Projects: Teaching Group Work Skills in a Distance-Learning Classroom" (Chapter 9) by Lonnie R. Helton and Edith M. Anderson describes the use of interactive television classrooms as one of the developing phenomena faculty and students have to learn to accept. Helton and Anderson present their study of teaching group work in such a setting, with two classes both divided between two different locations. The authors developed a group simulation project for each class and measured the outcomes for learning about group interaction and process, developmental stages, leadership roles, communication, power, etc. The students' learning is seen as positive, as is the faculty experience. In their review of literature and outcomes, Helton and Anderson note that much more investigation is needed to validate this interactive classroom approach for teaching group work, but their model for making use of the experience for the educational process gives us a good start.

"A Group Seminar to Enhance Field Instructors' Supervisory Skills" (Chapter 10) by Kathleen Holtz Deal describes how four three-hour seminars that involved experienced MSW field instructors evolved into a group process that led to sharing, support, and trust. This experience created increased "supervisory knowledge and skills through learning how to assess the normal stages of cognitive, affective, and behavioral development of MSW students and then tailor their supervision to fit their students' developmental learning needs." The authors identified and defined the characteristics of first-year MSW and second-year MSW students and recommended relevant approaches by field instructors to meet the learning needs of the students.

GROUP WORKERS FACING NEW AND UNPREDICTABLE SITUATIONS

Three very different situations called for rather unconventional approaches. "Yo no hablo Español: Facilitating a Group in Another Language" (Chapter 11) by Patricia M. Merle describes how six Mexican women came together to seek a better life. Two social workers from the United States had spent time in the area and had run workshops for women in prison. The Mexican women volunteered to oversee the work of a program sponsored by a U.S. church and sought help from the American social workers to become a group able to handle the tasks of their volunteer job and to support and nurture one another. The barrier was language. Communication took place despite barriers, with meaningful gains for both the Mexican and the American women. The clue for the social workers to reach their group members was in understanding and addressing what they value in their lives in a forbidding desert. They used the symbolism of "a rose grows in the desert" as a means to reinforce their sense of progress in what they were doing.

"'How Can I Talk About This Stuff?' Mutual Aid and Group Development in a Collectivity for Persons with Ulcerative Colitis" (Chapter 12) refers to the Pelvic Pouch Support Group, described by Catherine Coulthard, Joanne Sulman, and Brenda O'Connor. A Canadian university teaching hospital identified a need for a group to serve a vulnerable patient population—persons with ulcerative colitis. The group started out as a large, psychoeducational program and over time experienced issues of changing leadership, infrequent meetings, and large numbers of people who sporadically attended. In recognition of these group-relevant issues, the group is described as "a collective," a "social form," structured in such a way that becoming a group is precluded. The collectivity created a safe environment for sharing experiences, struggles, and suggestions. Although the Pelvic Pouch Support Group did not realistically become a group, it appeared to have a core subgroup and provided for a number of persons an opportunity to establish relationships outside the meetings. The need for support, relative to the unique medical situation, appeared to have been addressed.

Sarah Ann Schuh addresses the unusual situations faced by bone marrow transplant patients in "Efficacy of an Open-Ended Psychoeducational Support Group in a Health Care Setting" (Chapter 13). The program for bone marrow transplant (BMT) patients at the Fairview-University Medical Center in Minneapolis, Minnesota, recognized that a transplant is a physically, emotionally, and psychologically taxing procedure for both the patient and family. The social workers of the institution developed a group to provide support for patients' caregivers through education and peer support. The purpose of the group was to focus on the "psychosocial aspects of BMT, the hospital system, and community resources in order [to enhance] the patient's and family's functioning, [increase] their perceived sense of control, and [help] to reduce some of the anxiety that can detract from their participation in the patient's treatment." The group met weekly. It was designed as an open-ended psychoeducational support group that featured guest speakers and was the responsibility of the social workers. The group helped people cope with stress, trauma, and uncertainty associated with a bone marrow transplant.

INFORMING THE FUTURE

The final Plenary Session was in a group interactive format, with small-group discussions on the topic "Back to the Future: Envisioning Group Work Practice in Years to Come." It was facilitated by Marcia Cohen. Participants shared their hopes about group work practice models and social change via the group. What we envision for group work in the future, at a time of national crisis, thrust the participants into a reevaluation of the place of group work in this altered climate. Among "Our Hopes for the Future" were these reminders to ourselves "that we maximize the post-9/11 drift toward working with groups," and "at a time when the world is in crisis, we have to demonstrate basic group work values of social justice and mutual aid within tolerance of differences." The consensus was that the crises arising from the September 11 events had heightened our awareness of the importance of social action group work, now and in the future. Finally, we had a shared goal of ensuring the survival and growth of group work practice, informed by anti-oppressive and social change values and nurtured by the need of human beings to support one another.

PART I:
HISTORICAL PERSPECTIVES

Chapter 1

The Legacy of Ruby Pernell
and Social Group Work

Janice L. Andrews

INTRODUCTION

In many respects, this conference has as a major focus the celebra-
tion and honoring of the life and contributions of Dr. Ruby Pernell
(1917-2001). She would not approve. When Betty Lewis sent me the
obituary on Ruby from the *Cleveland Plain Dealer* (February 7,
2001), she noted that Ruby would not have liked all of the accolades,
but that she would have been "pleased that we loved her [because] respect is fine, but love is better" (personal communication, February
15, 2001). Ruby died this past February, just short of her eighty-
fourth birthday. She was working on the Twenty-Third International
AASWG Conference until shortly before her death.

She is remembered for her many gifts as a scholar, a true friend, a
listener, and a mediator. Alex Gitterman suggested that Ruby "will be
as close as we ever get to being with royalty . . . a colleague of uncommon dignity, class and style. . . . When Ruby spoke, we all listened"
(e-mail to AASWG board members, February 5, 2001). Katy Papell
added, "Ruby will [be] particularly remember[ed] . . . for her mediating wisdom. . . . Ruby quietly brought people together with a creative
suggestion for how to go on with the task at hand" (e-mail to John
Ramey, forwarded to AASWG board members, February 9, 2001).
Hans Eriksson remembers how inviting Ruby was to him and his
family during their stay in this country and how fortunate they were to
have Ruby stay with them in their home in Trondheim, Norway,
where she engaged the children in plays and activities (personal communication, February 28, 2001).

Betty Lewis referred to Ruby's ability to "let the process flow, to remain quiet and listen until the group needs some input to meld or compromise to a solution" (personal communication, August 7, 2001). As Lewis explained, much of Ruby's life was about "facilitating connections—bridging tender spots in such non-hostile or confrontive ways that we usually thought we'd done it ourselves. At the same time [she] enjoyed the power that she wielded when decisions went the way [she] suggested." It's not surprising that members of her family called her the "little general." Listening to Ruby, wrote Lewis, one would think "things just happened serendipitously and without planfulness on her part—the ultimate in group work skill."

Ruby did not like to talk about herself. When I asked her in 1999 if she would be willing to sit down with me for a series of interviews of her life for possible publication, she couldn't imagine anything in her life that could be of interest to others. She was a difficult interviewee. She had to be prodded to respond. When, early in the interview, I tried to pinpoint the circumstances of her family moving from Birmingham, Alabama, to Pittsburgh, Pennsylvania, she rather slowly replied, "I really didn't like [Birmingham], so I left when I was three weeks old!" Later, when I asked her to talk about the racial situation regarding housing in the Minneapolis/St. Paul community in the 1940s (knowing from Gisa Konopka that Ruby had struggled to find housing and that she lived with the Konopkas for some time after arriving at the University of Minnesota), Ruby wanted to know what I meant by "the racial situation." "Well," I meant, "for example, how segregated was the community?" She insisted:

> I didn't have any problem. I know that when I was going to move into the apartment . . . one of the neighbors came across the street to speak to [the landlord] to protest the idea [but] later she rented her garage to me and became a great supporter. (Pernell, in Andrews, 2001, p. 41)

A common response during the interviews was, "I don't initiate things; good things happen to me" or "Oh, I didn't do much" or "Really, it was a nothing job" (Pernell, in Andrews, 2001, p. 41). She told me that she has always been a very private person. A reporter at a Pittsburgh newspaper carried a story on Ruby when, in 1963, she was appointed as a social welfare attaché to the U.S. embassy in India. "Miss Pernell is an exceedingly modest person who avoids publicity," the writer noted. A sister of Ruby's, however, was very willing to discuss Ruby with the newspaper and shared that "[Ruby] turned down a number of foreign assignments mainly . . . because she took time to think them over. But this job developed so suddenly, she hadn't time to think too long" (Johnson, 1963).

PERNELL'S VITAE

Ruby Pernell was the Grace Longwell Coyle Professor Emerita at Case Western Reserve University. She was a major contributor to social group work knowledge, values, and skills for over fifty-five years through her work at Soho Community House; through her participation on numerous boards and committees around the globe, her teaching at the University of Minnesota and Case Western Reserve, as well as visiting professorships at the University of Denver, Atlanta University, and the University of Washington, Seattle; and through her training workshops and short courses in, to name a few countries, Britain, Jamaica, India, Germany, Canada, and Sri Lanka. She published and presented widely on group work, social development, policy, youth, and international understanding. She was one of the organizers of the first annual symposium of AASWG in 1979 in Cleveland and was active in AAGW from the mid-1940s. Throughout her career, she served as a board member on all of the major social work organizations in the United States and on many in other countries.

Ruby's BS (1939) and MSW (1944) were earned at the University of Pittsburgh. During a sabbatical leave in the 1950s, she got her PhD (1959) at the London School of Economics.

From Camping, YWCA, Urban League, to Social Work

When Ruby graduated from college, paying jobs were not plentiful and she took whatever she could find to support her. She spent her most pleasurable time doing volunteer work. She was active in Girl Reserves and loved camping. Her eventual desire to become a group worker was linked to her passion for camping. "I went to camp [one] summer [in the 1930s]," she explained:

> [T]hey had tried an experiment to see if it was alright to have
> "colored" girls at camp, so there were three or four of us. . . .
> Camp was so important to me. . . . We had a YWCA day camp,
> then we had Pittsburgh day camp, and I worked in both as a vol-
> unteer, and then from that into an overnight camping situation
> that the Urban League was starting [and] from that into graduate
> school. (Pernell, in Andrews, 2001, p. 36)

The Urban League camp focused on African-American history
and provided role models for the campers. The counselors were generally African-American college students (Pernell papers). Her early
involvement with the YWCA also fostered her increasing interest in
international affairs, which remained a lifelong passion.

Graduate studies at the University of Pittsburgh School of Social
Work in the early 1940s were exhilarating and stimulating for Ruby:
she named Gertrude Wilson, Gladys Ryland, Wilbur Newstetter,
Marion Hathway, and Margaret Berry as some of the faculty. There
was a very progressive orientation at Pittsburgh in general; social
group work added another dimension to the mix. Ruby explained:

> I think that group work, not in terms of political, but in terms of
> a kind of a cultural openness in orientation, . . . of that period
> was a marvelous kind of experience to really develop a liberal
> point of view, because we were still very much aware of and in-
> volved with settlements and their historical role and with the de-
> velopment of the Federation of Social Agencies, community
> councils, things of this sort that kept you related to the commu-
> nity; and because of where the settlement ethnic neighborhoods
> were got you aware of the cultural backgrounds of different peo-
> ple [and] the music, the dances. (Pernell, in Andrews, 2001,
> p. 37)

Classmates, some in her class, others overlapping, included Gisela
Konopka, Miriam Cohn, Bill Berry, Ruth Middleman, Celia Weisman, Bessie Pine, Helen Northen, Mary Lee Nicholson, Margaret
Hartford, Patricia Collins, Dorothy Bodin, and, later, Betty Lewis and
Hal Lewis. "Practically all of us became sort of [the] second generation of teachers" (Andrews, 2001, p. 39). She told of an instance
when she and Gisela were in Atlantic City at the National Conference
on Social Welfare:

We were walking down the boardwalk with some of our students and we met Gertrude Wilson and Gertrude says, "Oh, are these the grandchildren?" Since we were the children, our students were the grandchildren. . . . [I]t was just at the point where group work was developing at other schools. (Pernell, in Andrews, 2001, p. 38)

Ruby acknowledged that this cohort of students from Pittsburgh played an important role in the future of social group work:

I think we had a very great impact on group work. We had as great an impact on group work, I think, as the first generation because we were a direct line. In other words, what we were teaching and practicing at that point was what we had learned. (Pernell, in Andrews, 2001, p. 39)

Ruby found Gertrude Wilson to be an inspiration and was in awe of her and other early group workers. Ruby's field instructor shared with Ruby that Gertrude Wilson once complained about Ruby, "She just sits there like a sponge; soaking it all up!" (Pernell, 1992, p. 133).

PERNELL'S CAREER

After graduation, Ruby worked as the program coordinator at Soho Community House in Pittsburgh until, encouraged by her close friend Gisela Konopka, she accepted a teaching position at the University of Minnesota in the group work concentration. While at the University of Minnesota, she traveled widely and was a consultant on group work for youth in Germany in 1951, not long after the war. She made friends there who remained friends for the rest of her life.

The U.S. State Department arranged for consultants from the United States to teach working with groups using a democratic process in various schools in Germany. Ruby worked at a school in Bavaria and also did a month's course in Berlin with staff members from all of the schools. Several of the German youth leaders in the program later came to the University of Minnesota for their MSW degrees. At first it was very stressful for Ruby because of some hostility toward the Americans. She experienced a very powerful breakthrough with one group that exemplified the power of mutual aid and democratic participation. She explained:

> When we started out, it was our [the Americans'] problem—the content was constantly challenged. Then, it was the "other people" who were the problem. . . . At the end I was doing a summary and using the blackboard and then we had a break. There were a bunch of them gathered around the blackboard. They showed us what they had done. They had this diagram. "Here we are over here and here is this boat on the sea and just when we get straight and we know what we're doing, you're gone." They had moved from "their" fault to "ours." We're the ones [the Germans] responsible for what happened. It was lovely. (Pernell, in Andrews, 2001, p. 42)

Her sabbatical in the 1950s to London was not originally intended to result in any sort of a degree. She wanted to go abroad to experience being a "foreigner." She hoped it would help her be more sensitive to issues that foreign students had in the United States, but then she decided to combine intentions and also take some courses. She insisted:

> It really was my stupidity that led to my getting a degree, not my smarts. . . . [I]t was one of the most frustrating experiences of my life. I think that part of that frustration was that it yielded something positive. I felt it should not have been because it was less than I wanted. . . . What made this so terribly frustrating was that I was accorded too much respect. . . . So, that's what I fell into when I wanted to be treated as a blank slate. [I wanted to be treated like] a know nothing student. (Pernell, in Andrews, 2001, p. 43)

The sabbatical ended after one year, but, by now, she felt "trapped" into the doctoral program so she stayed an additional year. By the end of two years, Ruby had earned a PhD at the London School of Economics. Again, Ruby saw this as an example of how good things just keep happening to her.

Ruby left the University of Minnesota in 1963 (press release, August 6, 1963) when she was appointed social welfare attaché to the U.S. embassy in New Delhi, India. She was unsure of the job at first because she "wasn't sure the government and [her] could mix because [she] tended to be a free spirit" (Pernell, in Andrews, 2001, p. 44). The position of embassy social welfare attaché involved developing and maintaining contacts with social welfare agencies in India and interpreting these programs to relevant U.S. contacts. In addition, the attaché promoted a better understanding of U.S. social policy and objectives in the whole field of social welfare (University of Minnesota press release, 1963).

She found that the job gave her a great deal of latitude to be creative in her role as a sort of liaison between the two countries. She loved India and its people and found that social work was deep in the Indian tradition. This tradition was well established in Hindu, Moslem, and Christian communities. Both religiously and politically, "social work had meaning to care about the poor and destitute" (Pernell, in Andrews, 2001, p. 44). Indira Gandhi was the chairperson of the Indian Child Welfare Council while Ruby was in India. It was a powerful council and, thus, provided some additional clout to social work issues.

When the position was eliminated in 1968, Ruby was asked to accept the position of the Grace Coyle Chair at Case Western by Herman Stein, Dean of the School of Social Work, who happened to be on a mission in India at the time. After declining the offer at first, she finally accepted and began her new life in Cleveland.

In many respects, it was a paradoxical time for group workers. Sonia and Paul Abels (1981) have referred to this time in social work as the "generocide of social group work" (p. 10). On the one hand, group workers, in general, had strong identification with the profession of social work and were engaged in instituting what became known as the integrated, or generalist, perspective. They were, all in all, supportive of a close link with social work. This link provided a sense of professional prestige. On the other hand, there was mounting concern that group work was being shortchanged and swallowed up. Some questioned whether group work as a discrete entity would survive in the curriculum despite its core importance. Ruby remembered the arguments and the passion surrounding them:

> At one point I remember being absolutely furious . . . when I realized that, despite the fact that the chair of the masters program had a group work background, and the chair of the curriculum committee had a group work background, they had agreed on

the elimination of the group process course as a requirement. I was so angry. (Pernell, in Andrews, 2001, p. 46)

She retired in 1983 from Case Western; she continued writing and speaking on social group work as well as working as a volunteer in a hospice and with AASWG both locally and internationally. A review of her papers and presentations tell us what she found important.

SOME THEMES

Many of Ruby's speeches and professional papers began with a definition of terms. Words were important to her; they had precise meaning and should be used carefully. In "Empowerment and Social Group Work" (Pernell, 1986a), she spends twelve illuminating pages carefully dissecting the word *empowerment.* She looks at the word *power:* the ability or capacity to act or perform effectively. Then she reviews the word *empowered:* the capacity to influence the forces that affect one's life space for one's own and others' benefit. From there, she tells us about *social group work:* a method with the potential for achieving these qualities.

Ruby believed that the international dimension of social welfare programs and problems should be an integral part of social work education, both in academic study and experiential learning (Pernell, 1971). Regardless of her topic, she looked at it from an international perspective, using a lens that explored social and economic class as well as ethnic and racial variables. For example, she often lectured on youth. She had that rare ability to both individualize and categorize— an ability that many advocate, but few attain. While recognizing that the category *youth* has merit, she emphasized—at the same time— that more-advantaged youth are able to stay in the protective environment of the young into their midtwenties, while less-advantaged youth, by ages twelve through fifteen, are thrown into adulthood. She also pointed out that nations vary regarding ages of childhood, youth, and adulthood. In some countries, youth as young as twelve through fourteen are out of school and working full-time. Also, female youth and male youth have different meanings across different cultures and countries. The term cannot be generalized. She added that youth whose needs are not met inevitably protest. This "deviance" among youth in lower classes and youth of color is labeled *delinquent,* while similar protest, or "deviance," among middle- and upper-class white youth is called a *youth movement.*

Ruby was particularly concerned about the history of social group work. She wanted people to understand what happened when group work merged into NASW in 1955 and how what happened has affected group work today. Her goal was to see the ideals of social group work reestablished in practice. She acknowledged that "social group workers made a historic decision about their identification and affiliation and let go the identifiable bonds with recreation and informal education" (Pernell, 1986b, p. 13). A result was that social group work moved closer to a problem-oriented philosophy and problem-oriented agencies and away from more leisure time activities and more recreational agencies. "[T]he richness of the varied membership we'd had before" the merger was now gone, she noted (Pernell, in Andrews, 2001, p. 47).

Ruby referred to social group work and NASW as "the troubled marriage" at the AASWG symposium in 1994 and explained:

> [W]ith few exceptions group work had never been accepted by social work as a fully "professional" activity. Our propensity for play made us suspect. What was "play therapy" in the child guidance clinic was just "playing around" in the settlements. Even when caseworkers discovered that working with clients in groups might have some value, they did not turn to their professional colleagues, social group workers, for practice theory and models, but outside the profession to psychiatrists and family therapists. . . . It was ironic that just when caseworkers were discovering potentials of working with "health" and coping, group workers, despite their history, were focused on "illness" and dysfunction. It is not what casework or NASW did to us in this realm but what we did to ourselves. (Pernell, 1994, p. 11)

She believed that NASW "sucked us in and swallowed us; it used our organizational skills and leadership and ignored our professional claims" (1994, p. 13). Yet, by 1999, she had this "feeling that history repeats itself." She said:

> I'm not even sure it's a feeling. I think that, in a way, it's a fact that things come around again. Some of the kinds of emphases that we had early on in social group work are reappearing. I par-

ticularly think of socialization as a concern. I also think that it's interesting that so much of what was unique to social group work is now part of many other professional activities. (Pernell, in Andrews, 2001, p. 47)

For Ruby, one of the most important moments for social group work in the past thirty years was the rebirth of a group work organization in 1979: the Association for the Advancement of Social Work with Groups. She believed that the history of group work "is one that shows us in a way that we're not unique enough to preserve our identity within a large organization." The challenge for AASWG, in her view, is "whether or not to try to preserve a core of what has been called 'social group work' with its broader value commitments than necessarily lie in a variety of social work activities with groups." Here, she meant, "for example, value commitments to democratic process and a sense of responsibility that leads to social action. Also, it includes the emphasis on helping groups function in a simultaneous personally and socially satisfying way." Early on, social group work was doing both: working with the individual and with the group as a whole. What happened with the individual and what happened with the group were totally interrelated. She was concerned that we no longer teach that in our social work programs. She was worried that people no longer have the

> sense of this wider potential for the way in which one can be effective within the kind of society that we have. We have bundles of techniques to do this or to do that without this kind of sense of mission which . . . was part of the earlier education for social group work. (Pernell, in Andrews, 2001, p. 47)

Ultimately, what she wanted to underscore is that "there is more to 'social group work' than there is to 'social work with groups'." She insisted that these two terms are not synonymous, that social work with groups has a "much broader application," but social group work has a "depth dimension" that the other doesn't. In social group work the democratic dimension occurs through small-group activity. Part of the reason, from Ruby's perspective, that the AASWG board, of which she was a member, has struggled with the purpose of the social action committee is that it has not been approached from a social group work perspective. If it had been, the board would understand that clinical group work, social group work, and community group work can all exist in one group experience (Andrews, 2001, p. 47).

Ruby was very excited about the possibilities for social group work in the current sociopolitical climate. She was optimistic that the concepts would continue to survive and even thrive. In her typical spirit of hope for the future, she believed that

> AASWG and the times we live in provide us with the opportunity to rekindle the flame. [A turning wheel] does more than turn. When in contact with the ground it moves forward. Social group work, with its values, methods, and skills, is the wheel. The social milieu the ground which changes over time. There is something familiar about the ground we're on now. The needs for socialization, growth and enhancement have become apparent again as has the need for democracy, tolerance and action. . . . Group work as we *knew* it is newly relevant. (1994, p. 13)

IN CLOSING

Ruby told me about a group work meeting she attended in Cleveland in the 1940s while she was a graduate student. She went into

> this crowded room where these group work "greats" were holding forth debating whether their organization, the Association for the Study of Social Group Work, should become a membership organization. [She and other students] were sitting on the floor because there wasn't any other place to sit and looking at Grace Coyle and some of these "greats" [they had] read about all of the time. [Ruby and the other students] were in awe. (Pernell, in Andrews, 2001, p. 38)

Ruby, that's how we felt when we began coming to AASWG meetings and saw you holding forth and talking about social group work. We learned from you a commitment to social group work as a method to encourage human understanding, compassion, and social action. We are in awe of you. Thank you for the beautiful dignity and calmness, the wisdom and strength, and, most of all, for letting us know you, if even for only a little while.

REFERENCES

Abels, S. and P. Abels (1981) (Eds.). *Social Work with Groups: Proceedings, 1979 Symposium.* Louisville, KY: Committee for the Advancement of Social Work with Groups.

Andrews, J. (2001). A narrative interview with social group worker Ruby Pernell. *Reflections,* Summer, pp. 34-48.

Johnson, T. (1963). Dr. Ruby B. Pernell becomes attaché in Indian embassy. Ruby Pernell Collection, Social Work History Archives, University of Minnesota.

Pernell, R. (1971). *International perspectives on social work: Implications for social work education in the United States.* Invitational paper given at the annual meeting of the Council on Social Work Education.

Pernell, R. (1978). *Youth in international perspective.* Keynote address given at the First Annual Gisela Konopka Lecture Series. Minneapolis: University of Minnesota.

Pernell, R. (1979). *Purpose in social group work: A life model.* Paper given at the First Annual Symposium, Social Work with Groups, Cleveland, Ohio.

Pernell, R. (1986a). Empowerment and social group work. In Parnesk, M. (Ed.), *Innovations in Social Group Work.* Binghamton, NY: The Haworth Press, pp. 107-117.

Pernell, R. (1986b). Old themes for a new world. In Glaser, P. and N. Mayadas, *Group Workers at Work: Theory and Practice in the 80s.* Totowa, NJ: Rowman and Littlefield, pp. 11-21.

Pernell, R. (1992). Gertrude Wilson. *Journal of Teaching in Social Work* 6(2), 131-135.

Pernell, R. (1994). *Social group work and NASW: The troubled marriage.* Invitational paper given at the XVIII AASWG Symposium, Hartford, Connecticut.

Pernell papers. Ruby Pernell Collection. Social Welfare History Archives, University of Minnesota. (*Note:* These papers are part of the Social Group Work Collection established by the AASWG under the leadership of the late Celia Weisman.)

Chapter 2

Contributions of Research to Group Work

Helen Northen

Practice with groups is an art in the sense that it provides opportunities for helping clients through a caring relationship and creativity. But effective group work occurs only as the use of oneself is integrated with scientific knowledge derived from research in the behavioral and social sciences, related professions, and, most important, social work practice. Social workers have an ethical responsibility to understand and use the best available knowledge about practice with groups. This chapter summarizes examples of research on group work that contribute to successful outcomes for members.

Prior to the development of formal education for group work in universities, leaders in group service agencies sought relevant knowledge about groups and ways to help participants to achieve their goals in groups, with the functions of education, recreation, character building, or social action. They turned to what little research there was in sociology, psychology, progressive education, and social casework in order to discover useful information about problem solving, methods of group discussion, differential values of activities, and principles of informal education.

Formal education for group work originated in a university in 1923, largely through the influence of Wilbur Newstetter. He was director of a neighborhood center in Cleveland, Ohio, who believed that work with groups required professional education, which should be based on scientific knowledge. He convinced the dean of the School of Applied Social Sciences at Western Reserve University to establish a Group Service Training Course in 1923. He had a master's degree in sociology, with a special interest in small groups and communities. The name of the program was changed to Social Group Work in 1926 to ally it to Social Case Work, the other specialization in the school. In her history of the group work program, Margaret Hartford (1981) noted that under Newstetter's leadership, "an atmosphere of scientific inquiry permeated the school" (p. 99).

EARLY DEVELOPMENTS

To develop a scientific knowledge base, Newstetter established University Settlement as a laboratory for the study of group work. It was the first university-operated social work training center. Also, along with Wilbur Newstetter, Mark Feldstein, and Theodore Newcomb (1938), he began an experimental research project at Camp Wawokiye in 1926. It was a study of the interpersonal relations among boys who were referred to the camp from a Child Guidance Clinic for the purpose of improving their peer relationships. The researchers developed concepts about the process of acceptance-rejection that occurs in group interaction. They found that the children's needs could be met and their relationships improved through group association. They demonstrated that experimental research could be done in natural settings. Think of that: this early research dealt with both process and outcome.

When Newstetter was conducting his research, other faculty members were developing knowledge about groups as they are used in social work, through preparing and analyzing records of practice. The first major contribution was made by Clara Kaiser, who had joined the faculty in 1927. She taught group work courses and developed fieldwork placements for students at University Settlement. One of her major projects was creating methods for recording group process that could be used to discover and analyze values concepts, and principles of practice. That work resulted in the publication of *The Group Records of Four Clubs* in 1930.

Kaiser left Western Reserve University in 1934 to pursue advanced studies, and Grace Coyle was appointed to that position. Her famous book, *Social Process in Organized Groups,* had been published in 1930. It was her doctoral dissertation in sociology from Columbia University. Through content analysis of literature and documents of organizations, she offered a framework of concepts for understanding groups and their environments. When she arrived at Western Reserve University, one of her first projects was a follow-up of Kaiser's work on records of practice, resulting in the publication of *Studies in Group Behavior* in 1937. That book provided a framework of knowledge for understanding the structure and process of groups, utilizing case studies. Thus, early faculty used both experimental and case study methods of research in the development of theories of practice.

Beginning in the 1940s, major research consisted of identifying and analyzing major concepts about groups from publications in the social sciences and psychology, and testing their application to social work practice. Considerable attention was given to knowledge about differences in ethnicity, race, religion, social class, and gender and how to use that knowledge in practice (Wilson and Ryland, 1949). It was also the time when the application of selected aspects of psycho-analytic theory, especially ego psychology, was furthered by the work of Gisela Konopka (1963), Fritz Redl and David Wineman (1951, 1952), Saul Scheidlinger (1952), and Gertrude Wilson and Gladys Ryland (1949). More recently, numerous studies have been conducted on group processes and their implications for practice. Mary Louise Somers (1957), for example, identified and summarized the existing four group theories. Margaret Hartford published her book *Groups in Social Work* in 1971, in which she set forth knowledge about small groups, based primarily on social science research. She also demonstrated its use in social work. Charles Garvin brought that knowledge up to date in 1987.

GROUP DEVELOPMENT

Since the mid-1960s, considerable research has dealt with the ways that groups change over time and differences in interventions by social workers in each stage of development. The identification of stages in a group's development provides clues for assessing individual and group functioning and for selecting appropriate content and interventions. Interest in theories of group development occurred as early as 1949 when Gertrude Wilson and Gladys Ryland wrote that the group worker "affects the social process for the purpose of helping the action to move forward in relation to the interests and needs of the members" (p. 61). Gordon Hearn's (1957) article on the process of group development influenced social workers to give specific attention to changes in structure, goals, relationships, problems, and interactional processes that occur in groups over time. In an early article, Northen (1957) traced changes in the development of groups composed of disturbed adolescents from the initial selection of members through termination. But it was not until 1965 that the famous article by James Garland, Hubert Jones, and Ralph Kolodny from Boston identified and described stages, based on an analysis of social science research and their studies of groups of children and adolescents in community agencies.

James Whittaker (1970) compared several formulations of group development that had been published since the first one. He concluded that the model by Garland, Jones, and Kolodny represented the most complete statement to date on the subject and contained the basic elements of the other models. More recently, Linda Schiller (1995) studied records of groups of women, from which she formulated what she called a relational model. She found that members establish "a sense of safety in their group affiliations before they are able to take on and challenge each other" (p. 31). In still another study, Sylvia Zamudio (1998) found that, in closed and time-limited groups for bereaved boys and girls, ages eleven to fifteen, the groups developed in ways that were similar to Schiller's model. Recently, too, Toby Berman-Rossi (1992) and Berman-Rossi and Timothy Kelly (1998) contributed knowledge from their research. Despite some different emphases, it is clear that a major task for social workers is to pay attention to changes in a group's development and to intervene in ways that help the members move forward toward the achievement of their goals.

THE PLANNING PROCESS

The group's development is influenced by the nature and extent of planning that occurs prior to the group's first meeting. Roselle Kurland's research (1978) was based on a content analysis of the literature and interviews with teachers of group work. She found that, within agency and social contexts, six dimensions need to be considered in planning for the formation of a group:

1. *Need:* the problems, issues, and areas of concern of the prospective member
2. *Purpose:* the objectives of the group as a system, related to the goals of each member
3. *Composition:* the areas of homogeneity and heterogeneity that govern the selection of members for the group
4. *Structure:* the arrangements that facilitate the conduct of the group, including duration of service and the time, length, frequency, and place of meetings
5. *Content:* the means used, such as activities or discussion, to achieve the group's purpose
6. *Pregroup contact:* ways of contacting prospective members to determine the group's suitability for them and, if suitable, preparing them for membership

Some research has been conducted on each of these dimensions. Hartford (1971) reviewed the research on group purpose and goals, composition, size of groups, space, time, and open or closed groups. Diane Meadow (1992) conducted a controlled experiment with a sample composed of sixteen groups whose members had not had pregroup interviews with an equal number who had them. She concluded that pregroup interviews were successful in facilitating attendance and developing clarity of purpose and expectations but did not enhance risk-taking behaviors and cohesion.

GROUP PURPOSE

Within the planning process, research has dealt with the importance of clarifying the group's purpose and goals for each member. Evidence supports the proposition that harmony between the goals of individuals and the general purpose of the group enhances both the satisfaction of the members and the effectiveness of the group. Charles Garvin (1969), based on his research, found that early knowledge of the goals and expectations of members helps workers to understand the group interaction and to anticipate the degree of investment that members will have in the group. When workers perceived accurately the members' expectations, their responses tended to be more appropriate and there was significantly more movement into problem solving than in instances in which workers did not perceive the expectations correctly. He concluded that clarity of purpose contributes to achievement of goals. Similarly, N. Leonard Brown's (1971) research indicated that early exploration of expectations leads to congruence between workers and members in their attitudes toward the group. His conclusion was that developing mutual expectations as early as possible is significantly related to the effectiveness of group functioning and the satisfaction of members.

Social workers often find it difficult to present clearly, simply, and explicitly their view of the group's purpose. Hartford (1962) found that group workers frequently failed to make explicit the purpose or they intervened inappropriately in the process of formulating goals. When that happened, there was a tendency for the group not to form. Separate studies by Scott Briar (1966) and Florence Lieberman (1968) found that clients are more apt to continue in treatment when they and their workers share similar expectations of the goals. In such situations, there tends to be regular attendance, few dropouts, and high degrees of cohesiveness.

Clarity about goals by both workers and members and, more important, congruence between these perceptions are achieved in early meetings of groups. From their research, both Florence Clemenger (1965) and Marjorie Main (1964) discovered that the ability of social workers to perceive accurately each member's own goals and to use that knowledge in the planning process varied for different members. Some workers tended to stereotype certain members or to overlook isolates and other less-active members. These findings suggest that it is necessary to pay attention to each individual as well as the developing group system. Individualization becomes essential.

In their recent study of social work practice June Hopps, Elaine Pinderhughes, and Richard Shankar (1995) confirmed earlier findings that defining realistic expectations and setting high expectations were major contributors to positive outcomes.

SOCIAL RELATIONSHIPS

Enhancement of the quality of interpersonal relationships is a major purpose of social work with groups. Carl Rogers's (1957) famous research on what he called the therapeutic triad comprised a necessary condition for the success of counseling. The triad consists of empathic understanding, nonpossessive warmth, and genuineness or authenticity. Mary Russell (1990) reported that considerable evidence from research in psychology and psychiatry, as well as social work, lead to the conclusion that these qualities are a necessary condition for continuance in treatment and positive outcomes. Their importance, even when different theoretical models are used, was supported by Arthur Schwartz's (1977) comparative study of behavioral and psychodynamic models with two matched groups of clients. The major finding was that successful clients in both groups rated "the interpersonal interaction with the therapist as the single most important part of treatment" (p. 374). Nick Coady (1993) concluded from his study that the therapeutic alliance was one of the best predictors of outcome, regardless of the theoretical approach that was used, and Michel Mor-Barak (1991) described numerous studies that indicate "quite unanimously that social relationships are beneficial to health in a number of groups of people in varying situations" (p. 121). It is the quality of the relationships not only between individuals and their workers but also among the members that influences positive change.

CONTENT OF GROUPS

Content refers to the means groups use to achieve their purposes. It encompasses what is done, how it is done, and why it is done. Exploration with members about what they prefer to do or to discuss provides a natural base for understanding their primary concerns and their readiness to deal with particular issues. Aaron Rosen and Dina Lieberman (1972) studied the relevance of content to the experiences of members. The conclusion was that a clear mutual orientation between workers and clients in regard to the purpose assists workers in maintaining the focus on relevant content. In a study of two groups of adoptive parents, Martha Gentry's (1974) findings supported the importance of the worker's initiation and maintenance of an appropriate focus on the topics related to the purpose that the members felt to be important. Dropouts were often related to the extent to which the members' expectations about content were not met.

GROUP COHESION

Social workers make efforts to develop group cohesion, based on findings from research that cohesion has an important influence on the development of the group.

The concept refers to the attraction that members have for one another and for the group as an entity. Avraham Levy's (1984) summary of research on cohesion found that the more cohesive the group, the greater the positive influence it has on its members. However, strong cohesion can also have negative influences. Nancy Evans and Paul Servis (1980) found that that happens when cohesion becomes the ends, rather then the means toward achieving other goals. Groups vary in the degree to which members are attracted to one another and to the group as an entity.

CLUSTERS OF INTERVENTIONS

Interpersonal and group relationships, as discussed earlier, have been found to be crucial elements of practice with groups, but effective problem solving requires that social workers also need knowledge and skills in developing the group and intervening in the group process. How to describe the complex constellation of ways to help groups is a thorny problem. Authors use different terms to describe the set of interventions from which practitioners select a particular one, according to their cumulative understandings of the person-group-environment situation at a given time. These clusters of interventions are often referred to as techniques or skills. In spite of the differences in terms, there is considerable agreement about types of interventions used to achieve particular goals.

Francis Peirce (1966) based his research on the idea that each major action of the social worker is motivated by an intention. He found that the verbal and nonverbal actions of workers are intended to

1. support an individual, subgroup group system, or relevant persons in the environment;
2. enhance the clarity of members' modes of communication;
3. improve the accuracy of members' perceptions of reality;

4. enhance members' competence to master life experiences; and
5. modify the environment so it can support members in their efforts toward growth and change or so that destructive environmental stresses are reduced.

In a comparative study of socialization and therapeutic groups, Gideon Horowitz (1968) found that similar skills are used with both types of groups: they are generic.

Marian Fatout (1975) conducted a content analysis of major books and relevant research on practice to discover generic interventions. Based on her analysis and the research of Lawrence Shulman (1992) and Lynn Videka-Sherman (1988), it is suggested that the major clusters of skills are structuring, support, exploration, information/education, advice/guidance, confrontation, clarification, and interpretation (Northen, 1988). They are used both with members of groups and significant persons in the environment.

TERMINATION

Studies that have been done on termination deal primarily with the emotional reactions of the members to leaving the group or to the ending of the group. A group has been formed and sustained as members worked to achieve particular goals. Now, when faced with the loss of the worker and relationships with one another, the members react with a variety of emotions and behaviors. General agreement is found in the research on both socialization and psychosocial treatment groups that varied emotional reactions occur (Garland, Jones, and Kolodny, 1965; Northen and Kurland, 2001).

Benjamin Lewis (1978) studied fourteen therapy and ten socialization groups, predominantly composed of adolescents. The groups, led by practitioners with master's degrees in social work met weekly for an average of one year. The purpose of the research was to test the characteristics of the termination stage as formulated by Garland and associates (1965). The study confirmed the presence of major categories of emotional reactions of members, although not all groups exhibited all reactions. In her research, Mary Lackey (1981) also confirmed the presence of multiple emotional reactions to termination. In a content analysis of records of four groups of adults, she found many positive expressions about termination as well as a range of negative ones. She concluded that the conflict between the acknowledgment of improvement and fear of the loss of the worker's help and the group's support led to various strong feelings about the ending. Clearly, members need help to work through their ambivalence. In another study, Anne Fortune (1987) found that almost all members had some negative reactions to termination There were, however, more positive than negative ones. As members discussed their ambivalence, they were more likely to feel satisfied with the group experience.

EVALUATION OF RESULTS

The ultimate test of the effectiveness of group work practice is the extent to which the members have made positive changes in achieving their goals. Evaluation is complex. According to Robert Chin (1960, p. 42), "Evaluation studies of goal achievement are of limited importance unless the evaluation study also tries to pinpoint the components which 'cause' the degree of attainment or hindrance of goals." Thus, both process and outcomes need to be studied.

There is growing evidence from research that groups tend to be effective in achieving their purposes. In Ronald Toseland's and Max Siporin's (1986) major review of research, thirty-two studies were discovered that compared individual and group treatment and that used classic experimental designs with control groups, standardized measurements, and face-to-face contacts between clients and practitioners. The results were positive for both individual and group treatment, but in eight of the studies, group treatment was found to be significantly more effective than individual treatment. Fewer dropouts also occurred in groups. No clear pattern emerged concerning what types of clients or problems were best suited for groups. Other factors, such as the theoretical approach used and characteristics of the group's structure and process, may have influenced the findings. Of course, too, the differential competence of workers may be a factor.

Other reviews of research on outcome tend to confirm the findings of Toseland and Siporin (1986). Mary Russell's (1990) review of evaluation research on groups demonstrated that a variety of theoretical approaches were used, with therapy predominant. Positive findings were found, particularly in groups with a social support or mutual aid function and in structured groups in which specific problems were addressed. In another earlier review, Robert Dies (1983) concluded, "The results clearly support the efficacy of group treatment" (p. 5). In a recent study of clinical social work practice with overwhelmed clients, Hopps, Pinderhughes, and Shankar (1995) reported that, although social agencies preferred the one-to-one approach, group work offered a strong potential for changing the norms and behavior of overwhelmed clients, particularly youth and young adults. When groups were used, there was "success in overall functioning as demonstrated by movement in self esteem, self mastery, competence and enhanced differentiation" (p. 165). They were effective in helping members to focus action on urgent and pressing problems, such as drugs and violence in their neighborhoods. Still, not all people are helped through groups. Some may be harmed. Casualties do occur in groups, as Maeda Galinsky and Janice Schopler (1977) and Schopler and Galinsky (1981) found in their research.

Evaluation of practice is becoming more sophisticated in determining the relationship between outcomes and the nature and quality of practice. An example is that of a controlled experiment to compare the effectiveness of multifamily group therapy and traditional family therapy. The groups were composed of families in which abuse and/or neglect had occurred and in which there was at least one child between the ages of two and eleven. The researchers, William Meezan and Maura O'Keefe (1998), reviewed the relevant literature, described the plan for the group, set criteria for membership, made random assignments to an experimental or traditional family therapy group, developed measurable objectives, and made decisions about the content and structure of the groups. In evaluating outcomes, multiple measures of adult, child, and family functioning were used. The findings were that multifamily group therapy was a more effective approach in the treatment of abusing and neglecting families than was traditional family therapy.

CONCLUSIONS

From this all-too-brief review of examples of research on social work with groups, the conclusion is that studies have indeed contributed to understanding the nature and quality of practice. From its very beginnings, some leaders in education have strongly supported the need for scientific knowledge about groups: their structures, processes, and development, and the effectiveness of their use in social work with groups. The focus has been on the use of that knowledge to help members to achieve their desired goals related to the enhancement of psychosocial functioning. Much more needs to be done.

Ben Orcutt (1990) suggests that professional competence "evolves out of commitment, curiosity, and the thirst for knowledge—a creative, imaginative search to know." Group workers have an ethical responsibility to practice within the values of the profession of social work and the knowledge gained through analysis of experience and research. It can be exhilarating to realize that one has achieved success and know why that has happened (Northen and Kurland, 2001).

REFERENCES

Berman-Rossi, T. (1982). Empowering groups through stages of group development. *Social Work with Groups* 15(2-3), 239-256.

Berman-Rossi, T. and Kelly, T.B. (1998). *Advancing stages of group development theory*. Paper presented at the Forty-Fourth Annual Symposium, Association for the Advancement of Social Work with Groups.

Briar, S. (1966). Family services. In H.S. Maas (Ed.), *Five Fields of Social Service: Reviews of Research*, pp. 9-50. New York: National Association of Social Workers.

Brown, N.L. (1971). Social workers' verbal acts and the development of mutual expectations with beginning client groups. DSW dissertation, Columbia University.

Chin, R. (1960). Evaluating group movement and individual change. In National Association of Social Workers (Ed.), *Use of Groups in the Psychiatric Setting*, pp. 34-45. New York: NASW.

Clemenger, F. (1965). Comparison between members and workers on selected behaviors of the role of the social group worker. DSW dissertation, University of Southern California.

Coady, N. (1993). The worker-client relationship revisited. *Families in Society*, 74, 291-300.

Coyle, G.L. (1930). *Social Process in Organized Groups*. New York: Smith.

Coyle, G.L. (1937). *Studies in Group Behavior*. New York: Harper.

Dies, R. (1983). Bridging the gap between research and practice in group psychotherapy. In R.R. Dies and K.R. MacKenzie, *Advances in Group Psychotherapy*, pp. 1-26. New York: International Universities Press.

Evans, N. and Servis, P.A. (1980). Group cohesion: A review and re-evaluation. *Small Group Behavior*, 11(4), 359-370.

Fatout, M.F. (1975). Comparative analysis of practice concepts described in selected social work literature. DSW dissertation, University of Southern California.

Fortune, A.E. (1987). Grief only? Client and social worker reactions to termination. *Clinical Social Work Journal,* 15(2), 159-171.

Galinsky, M.J. and Schopler, J.H. (1977). Warning: Groups may be dangerous. *Social Work,* 22(2), 89-94.

Garland, J.A., Jones, H.E., and Kolodny, R.L. (1965). A model for stages of development in social work groups. In S. Bernstein (Ed.), *Explorations in Group Work,* pp. 17-71. Boston: Boston University School of Social Work.

Garvin, C.D. (1969). Complementarity of role expectations in groups: The member-worker contract. In National Conference on Social Welfare, *Social Work Practice,* 1969, pp. 127-145. New York: Columbia University Press.

Garvin, C.D. (1987). Group theory and research. In *Encyclopedia of Social Work.* Washington, DC: National Association of Social Workers.

Gentry, M. (1974). Initial group meetings: Member expectations and information distribution process. PhD dissertation, Washington University.

Hartford, M.E. (1962). The social group worker and group formation. PhD Dissertation, University of Chicago.

Hartford, M.E. (1971). *Groups in Social Work.* New York: Columbia University Press.

Hartford, M.E. (1981). The contributions of Grace Coyle and the faculty of the School of Applied Social Sciences of Western Reserve University to group practice theory. In S.L. Abels and Paul Abels (Eds.), *Social Work with Groups: Proceedings 1979 Symposium,* pp. 91-119. Louisville, KY: Committee for the Advancement of Social Work with Groups.

Hearn, G. (1957). The process of group development. *Autonomous Group Bulletin,* 13.

Hearn, G. (1958). *Theory Building in Social Work.* Toronto: University of Toronto Press.

Hopps, J., Pinderhughes, E., and Shankar, R. (1995). *The Power to Care.* New York: Free Press.

Horowitz, G. (1968). Worker interventions in response to deviant behavior in groups. PhD dissertation, University of Chicago.

Kaiser, C. (1930). *The Group Records of Four Clubs at the University Settlement Center.* Cleveland: School of Applied Social Sciences, Western Reserve University.

Konopka, G. (1963). *Social Group Work: A Helping Process.* Englewood Cliffs, NJ: Prentice-Hall.

Kurland, R. (1978). Planning: The neglected component of group development. *Social Work with Groups,* 1(2), 1-3.

Lackey, M.B. (1981). Termination: The critical stage of social work. DSW dissertation, University of Southern California.

Levy, Avraham (1984). Group cohesion. PhD dissertation, University of Southern California.

Lewis, B.F. (1978). An examination of the final phase of a group development theory. *Small Group Behavior,* 9(4), 507-517.

Lieberman, F. (1968). Clients' expectations, preferences and experiences of initial interviews in voluntary social agencies. DSW dissertation, Columbia University.

Main, M.W. (1964). Selected aspects of the beginning phase of social group work. PhD dissertation, University of Chicago.

Meadow, D. (1992). The effects of a client-focused pre-group preparation interview on the formation of group cohesion and members' interactional behavior. PhD dissertation, University of Southern California.

Meezan, W. and O'Keefe, M. (1998). Evaluating the effectiveness of multifamily group therapy in child abuse and neglect. *Research on Social Work Practice,* 8(3), 330-353.

Mor-Barak, M. (1991). *Social Networks and Health of the Frail Elderly.* New York: Garland.

Newstetter, W.I., Feldstein, M.J., and Newcomb, T.N. (1938). *Group Adjustment: A Study in Experimental Sociology.* Cleveland: Western Reserve University.

Northen, H. (1957). Evaluating movement of individuals in social group work. In *Group Work Papers 1957.* New York: National Association of Social Workers.

Northen, H. (1988). *Social Work with Groups.* New York: Columbia University Press.

Northen, H. and Kurland, R. (2001). *Social Work with Groups,* Third Edition. New York: Columbia University Press.

Orcutt, B.A. (1990). *Science and Inquiry in Social Work Practice.* New York: Columbia University Press.

Peirce, F.J. (1966). A study of the methodological components of social work with groups. DSW dissertation, University of Southern California.

Redl, F. and Wineman, D. (1951). *Children Who Hate.* Glencoe, IL: Free Press.

Redl, F. and Wineman, D. (1952). *Controls from Within: Techniques for the Treatment of the Aggressive Child.* Glencoe, IL: Free Press.

Rogers, C.R. (1957). The necessary and sufficient conditions of therapeutic personality change. *Journal of Consulting Psychology,* 21, 95-103.

Rosen, A. and Lieberman, D. (1972). The experimental evaluation of interview performance of social workers. *Social Service Review,* 46(3), 395-412.

Russell, M.N. (1990). *Clinical Social Work: Research and Practice.* Newbury Park, CA: Sage.

Scheidlinger, S. (1952). *Psychoanalysis and Group Behavior.* New York: Norton.

Schiller, L.Y. (1995). Stages of development in women's groups: A relational model. In Kurland, R. and Salmon, R. (Eds.), *Group Work Practice in a Troubled Society,* pp. 17-38. Binghamton, NY: The Haworth Press.

Schopler, J.H. and Galinsky, M.J. (1981). When groups go wrong. *Social Work,* 26(5), 424-429.

Schwartz, A. (1977). Behaviorism and psychodynamics. *Child Welfare,* 56(6), 368-379.

Somers, M.L. (1957). Four small group theories: An analysis and frame of reference for use in social group work. DSW dissertation, Western Reserve University.

Toseland, R.W. and Siporin, M. (1986). When to recommend group treatment: A review of the clinical and research literature. *International Journal of Group Psychotherapy,* 36(2), 171-206.

Videka-Sherman, L. (1988). Meta analysis of research on social wok practice in mental health. *Social Work,* 33(4), 325-338.

Whittaker, J.K. (1970). Models of group development: Implications for group work practice. *Social Service Review,* 44(3), 308-322.

Wilson, G. (1976). From practice to theory: A personalized history. In Roberts, R.W. and Northen, H. (Eds.), *Theories of Social Work with Groups,* pp. 1-44. New York: Columbia University Press.

Wilson, G. and Ryland, G. (1949). *Social Group Work Practice.* Boston: Houghton-Mifflin.

Zamudio, S. (1998). *Stages of group development in children's bereavement groups.* Paper presented at the Twentieth Annual Symposium, Association for the Advancement of Social Work with Groups, October.

Chapter 3

Group Work at Hull House: Lessons from the Past, Signposts for the Future

Diane C. Haslett

INTRODUCTION

Group work practitioners trace their roots to three sources: progressive education, the recreation movement, and the settlement movement (Rosenblatt and Waldfogel, 1983, p. 29). Hull House, Chicago's most famous settlement house, was central to the development of group work and provided the foundation for much of contemporary social work practice with groups. The ensuing discussion of the work of Rachelle Yarros, a physician who lived and worked at Hull House while building path-breaking programs in reproductive health, illustrates one aspect of early group work. Beyond historical interest, Yarros's example spurs today's group workers to reflect on the efficacy of current practice.

Early in their educational programs, social work students usually discover Jane Addams and the inner circle of Hull House residents in books, journals, and other articles (Addams, [1910] 1961; Carson, 1990; Costin, 1980; Davis and McCree, 1969; Eaton, 1894; Hamilton, [1943] 1985; Lissak, 1989; Mackevich, Ruoff, and Vavra, 1989; Sicherman, 1984; Wade, 1971). Most have likely never heard of Rachelle Yarros's work, which, while visionary and inventive, has received limited attention in the literature on Hull House (Bryan and Davis, 1990; Bryan, Slote, and De Angury, 1996; Johnson, 1990; Lasch, 1971; Mackevich, Ruoff, and Vavra, 1989; Polikoff, 1999; Sicherman, 1984; Stebner, 1997; Ward, 1986).

Furthermore, Hull House residents' involvement in the cause of birth control is generally overlooked or receives only passing comment in texts and articles on the Progressive Era (Carson, 1990; Chen, 1996; Chesler, 1992; Clarke, 1961; Ditzion, 1969; Gordon, 1977; Kennedy, 1970; Reed, 1978). This lack of attention persists despite the presence in the historical record of articles and other writings on the subject by the women of Hull House (Holmes et al., 1908; Hamilton, 1910, 1925, [1943] 1985; Hull-House Year Book, 1927; Kelly, 1919) and of the involvement of Jane Addams and Hull House in efforts to bring birth control information and services to Chicago (Addams, [1912] 1970; Hamilton, [1943] 1985; Haslett, 2001; Kennedy, 1970; Reed, 1978; Ward, 1990; Yarros, 1919b; Yarros, 1920). This chapter presents and analyzes Yarros's use of groups as vehicles for sex education and social reform in the community and at the policy level with particular emphasis on her work in primary prevention. It not only highlights her accomplishments as an important historical figure pioneering in reproductive health programs and education but also informs current group work practice in the fields of sex education, contraception, and reproductive freedom.

BACKGROUND

Like many who participated in Hull House programs, Rachelle Slobodinsky Yarros was an immigrant, exiled from the Ukraine because of her radical political activities. Her connection with members of the Hull House inner circle began in the early 1890s when she and Alice Hamilton were interns at New England Hospital for Women and Children in Boston (Sicherman, 1984). In a letter to Agnes Hamilton in 1893, Hamilton recounts Yarros's early days:

> Dr. Sloboda—as we have to call her for short—is the most interesting thing. . . . She is only our age, but she has lived through more than we will have when we are sixty. Yet through it all she is a light-hearted, natural girl. . . . Think! She began to be a Nihilist when she was thirteen years old. . . . Of course her parents were bitterly opposed to her doings, and no wonder, for the police used to come to her father every now and then, and tell him that, if he did not stop her going to those young people's clubs and talking so imprudently, they would simply have to arrest

her. Finally matters came to such a pass that it was a question between banishment of some kind and flying the country, so she decided to come to America. (Sicherman, 1984, pp. 65-66)

Yarros seemed destined for work in the settlement movement. At that time she told Hamilton that "the only way to reach the working classes is by living right among them" (Sicherman, 1984, p. 66), echoing Jane Addams's early words:

> On that day I had my first sight of the poverty which implies squalor. . . . I remember launching at my father the pertinent inquiry why people lived in such horrid little houses so close together, and that after receiving his explanation I declared with much firmness when I grew up I should, of course have a large house, but it would not be built among the other large houses, but right in the midst of horrid little houses like these. (Addams, [1910] 1961)

In 1897 Hamilton found her way to Hull House. Later she, too, became a vigorous advocate for birth control and a frequent contributor to the *Birth Control Review,* the monthly publication of Margaret Sanger's American Birth Control League. In 1907 Rachelle Yarros and her husband Victor, a journalist, followed, also becoming residents of Hull House and staying for twenty years (Lasch, 1971). While a Hull House resident, Yarros was also an associate professor at the College of Physicians and Surgeons of Chicago. As associate professor, she broke new ground in obstetrical education and in teaching about human sexuality and contraception. From 1898 to 1910 Yarros taught courses in obstetric care and home deliveries for classes of both male and female medical students in the college's Department of Obstetrics in the Ghetto, an approach rarely taken then. Teaching students in real-life conditions in the neighborhoods was a central tenet of her educational philosophy, similar to social work's field practicum for aspiring practitioners. In 1926 the University of Illinois College of Medicine awarded her a full professorship in social hygiene, in honor of her pioneering work in social hygiene and sex education (Ward, 1986).

Following a path already trod by Margaret Sanger in her career as a nurse in New York's Lower East Side (Sanger, [1938] 1971, pp. 86-92), Yarros was moved to action by the dreadful conditions in which her patients lived. She became a vocal advocate of the cause of birth control by joining with Sanger and others who challenged policies denying women and men access to information and contraceptive devices and by providing direct services such as neighborhood medical centers and day nurseries. Yarros harnessed the power of educational groups, using them to inform and to have impact on people's behavior, and the power of social action groups, using them to make significant institutional change. In current terms, her fight for birth control is a clear illustration of a systems approach to social reform in reproductive freedom through group work. As such, it continues to be relevant today.

WOMEN'S CLUBS AND THE MEDICAL CENTERS: GROUPS FOR CAUSE AND FUNCTION

Like many professional women of her day, Yarros was a member of several women's organizations. Her membership and influence with women's groups in Chicago and nationally helped to advance the twin causes of birth control and social hygiene. In her years at Hull House, Rachelle Yarros employed her earlier experience as a political activist in the Ukraine and a labor organizer in Rahway, New Jersey, to establish the Birth Control Committee of the Chicago Woman's Club (Sicherman, 1984; Yarros, 1919b, 1932a). Under her able leadership this committee later organized the Illinois Birth Control League. The immediate focus was on education. However, in 1922, answering the call of Margaret Sanger and responding to the needs Yarros daily encountered, those two groups and other individuals prominent in the birth control movement joined with Yarros to create Chicago's first, and the nation's second, public birth control clinic. The effort was stalled by the commissioner of health's refusal to grant the license. Not surprising, the courts sided with the commissioner even though Illinois law did not bar distribution of birth control information (Ward, 1990). This opposition only strengthened the group's resolve. The league opened a private clinic in the business district of Chicago, making the license unnecessary.

At their most productive, eight clinics served women in Chicago's neighborhoods. Mary Crane Nursery, another innovative Hull House program—this time in early childhood education—was the site of one clinic. This linkage was a significant early example of a multiservice, neighborhood-based agency serving the needs of mothers and their children (Yarros, 1925). Mary Crane Nursery exists today, although now relocated in Chicago's Lathrop Homes, a public housing development on the North Side. The clinic is no longer part of the nursery's service delivery system.

These clinics, which served several thousand women, many from lower socioeconomic groups, illustrate the unique blending of social work's dual emphasis on cause and function (Lee, 1929). The logical extension of advocating for birth control information and services was to provide those services through accessible clinics in the neighborhoods. These clinics were overwhelmingly successful. Data from 1929 (Yarros, 1931a) show that the six clinics then in operation provided contraceptive advice to 1,340 women, with 96 percent of the patients using a contraceptive method effectively from one to fourteen months. Besides providing concrete services to Chicago's families, data gathered from the clinics served as ammunition in refuting erroneous claims from the medical establishment about the supposed dangers of birth control (Yarros, 1931a). This approach, embedded in the Hull House tradition, exemplifies how the skillful worker moves among system levels from the organizational task group to provision of direct therapeutic services to creating institutional change based on research data from those direct services.

NATIONAL ORGANIZATIONS: CONFRONTING THE OPPOSITION

In her fight for quality reproductive health services, Yarros's style was characterized by vigorous activism and always involved work with organizational task groups. For example, she was a founder of the American Social Hygiene Association in 1914 and was the first vice president of the Illinois Social Hygiene League (Lasch, 1971; Ward, 1986). During World War I she chaired the Department of Social Hygiene of the Illinois State Council of Defense, extending her influence and impact to the state. Ultimately she gained prominence at the national level through her work for the American Birth Control League (Yarros, 1938a). Following World War I, she lectured frequently across the country for the national YWCA on topics relating to social hygiene (Yarros, 1919a).

Yarros published extensively in medical journals, social work periodicals, and in the American Birth Control League's *Birth Control Review.* Her articles demonstrate a well-honed ability to illustrate hard, statistical data with rich qualitative material reflecting the lives of the women and families served. Her daily experience in the clinics and her publications provided a strong base for Yarros as an authority on birth control, an attribute she used successfully in her various group encounters at both the micro and macro levels of practice (Yarros, 1925, 1931a,b). While most of her work was of a positive sort, Yarros was not afraid to use her authority and her leadership to confront organizations that attempted to undermine the cause of birth control and social hygiene. In a style worthy of a Chicago politician, Yarros used her "clout" in opposing the Chicago Medical Society's censure of Dr. Louis Schmidt of the Illinois Public Health Institute for his work in prevention and treatment of venereal disease in Chicago's neighborhoods. Yarros resigned her membership in protest and chastised the society for its reluctance to support the institute's efforts (Yarros, 1929).

SOCIAL REFORM: SEX EDUCATION
AND PREMARITAL COUNSELING

Yarros was in the vanguard of those supporting sex education for adolescents and worked to establish sex education programs in conjunction with Hull House and through the Illinois Social Hygiene Society. She fully understood the power of groups in working with young people. The methods she chose anticpated those used by sex educators today—lecture, discussion, small groups, and film. Yarros's description of the planning and implementation of these socio-educational groups provides a useful guide for primary prevention programming and a sound approach to group work intervention at the community level (Yarros, 1920, 1938, 1943).

Yarros believed that accessibility was central in the provision of effective services. She argued that young people would participate in these services if they were offered in locations young people frequented—religious institutions, their places of employment, Hull House programs, and the local Park District field houses where they spent their leisure time (Yarros, 1920, 1938, 1943). In a report to the Woman's City Club, Yarros (1920) outlined the strategies she used:

The question that confronted us was how to reach the various groups with the greatest certainty and in the largest numbers. In the city, the answer to this was the places where they work, study, gather for amusement and for club work. (p. 3)

Yarros had an acute understanding of systems and the dynamics involved in gaining cooperation from those in authority in the various host settings where she planned to implement her programs. In the same report she noted:

We found from experience that in order to secure permission to lecture in such establishments—*on the employers' time*—it was absolutely essential to send a competent person to interview first the one in charge of the group, and second, the employer himself in most cases. . . .

One of the most frequent objections made was lack of space for assemblage, but we found that whenever we convinced those in authority of the necessity, some place could always be found for the purpose.

A most interesting piece of work was done in banks. At first, the bank officials did not see why the type of girls they employed should have to be instructed in such matters. They were, however, persuaded to send a representative to hear one of the lectures, and as a result we gave ten talks in banks, reaching approximately 800 girls. (Yarros, 1920, p. 6)

Accommodation to the needs of the host setting is illustrated by Yarros's comments on how she adapted the program to suit the bank and office venues. When the number of employees was too large for them to be released at the same time without interrupting the work, Yarros and her staff staggered several small-group sessions to adapt the program to office routines (Yarros, 1920, p. 7).

Follow-up contacts were essential to the success of the programs. Yarros (1920) showed insightful use of attractive program strategies in her description of the film, a relatively new invention at that point, to help ensure attendance at the follow-up event:

As a piece of follow-up work, the girls were invited later to attend a showing of "The End of the Road" film (which was shown twice in order to accommodate all of them), arranged immediately after working hours. . . . An opportunity was given to the girls to ask questions. The interest in the subject proved to be very keen. (p. 7)

Furthermore, Yarros's approach exemplified formative evaluation at its best. She and her colleagues used their observations to fine-tune and improve their program to suit the needs of potential group members and increase program effectiveness.

She was also aware of the importance of gaining the approval of an influential member of the target community, in this case a large school. The influence of officials at the first school was central to the expansion of the program to other schools:

The more we worked with business girls, the more we realized we ought to try to reach the girl and talk to her about these matters before she entered on a business career. . . . Here again the managers of the schools hesitated, wondering whether they had the right to introduce such education. Finally one of the largest schools was persuaded to give us a chance, and after this first entrance it was comparatively easy to secure the consent of the other schools. (Yarros, 1920, p. 7)

These programs were remarkably well received. In her account to the Woman's City Club, Yarros (1920) reported that 661 lectures were given in Illinois, with 478 delivered in Chicago, reaching a total of 73,388 individuals, primarily women and girls. Considering that the efficacy of sex education faces challenges and opposition even now, Yarros's work was impressive. Her ability to gain allies in the established institutions of the day is clear from the support she received from the Chicago Church Federation and other Chicago civic groups and organizations, including the Chicago Public Schools.

In alliance with the educational division of the Illinois Social Hygiene League, Yarros opened the first Midwestern premarital and marital counseling service in 1932. Here again she employed her skill in working with task groups, this time with the Illinois Social Hygiene League, as she created yet another opportunity to provide primary prevention services and expanded her work in sex education in a new direction (Yarros, 1932b).

In 1938, Julius-Haldeman reprinted a low-cost version of Yarros's 1933 book *Modern Women and Sex,* retitled *Sex Problems in Modern*

Society (Yarros, 1938b). With the publication of this volume, she reached the culmination of her educational work by providing this information to the larger community. Yarros wished this information to be accessible to everyone interested, even those who might "not be in a position to pay $2 for any educational work, even if they feel keenly their need of it" (Yarros, 1938b, Preface).

IMPLICATIONS FOR SOCIAL WORK PRACTICE WITH GROUPS

Yarros's work with groups in the community and on the state and national levels illustrates a systems approach to education, primary prevention, and social reform that is well worth recognition and study. She understood and addressed the intricate issues interwoven with sex education, birth control, and reproductive health. She saw that the etiology of poverty, women's issues, classism, and ethnocentrism were all tied to the issues of birth control. Furthermore, she knew that these issues should be handled differently at each system level and that groups were a prime way to create the changes she envisioned. Yarros grasped and employed sound group work principles in her work with both socioeducational and social action groups. She worked with both types of groups to create social change at multiple system levels from the small discussion group at Hull House to larger groups in host settings to committee groups within local, regional, and national organizations. Yarros was adept at creating links across organizations to multiply the effectiveness and the scope of her work, offering a fine example of networking as relevant now as in her day.

Moreover, Yarros understood the need for comprehensive delivery of services, from sex education for youth to premarital/marital counseling and culminating with birth control clinics accessible even to working mothers. She knew that providing supportive services at each stage of a woman's sexual life and reproductive journey was and is essential in a just and caring society.

Yarros also understood the need for research to undergird practice. She learned well from her years at Hull House and used the empirical evidence from her day-to-day practice to improve services and to promote social change. Based on clinic records and practice experience, her documentation of the deleterious effects of multiple pregnancies and the significant costs of prohibiting abortion illustrates her approach to reform on the micro and macro levels. The connections between research and practice and the responsibility of social workers to provide systematic data to support social change are evident in Yarros's example. She perceived, understood, and used the link between what she learned in her work with individuals and small groups and her work for social change.

Considering that Yarros held and voiced some highly controversial views and that she was not an integral part of the better-known Hull House inner circle, it is not surprising that scholars have not explored her work more fully. However, the time has come to highlight her work as part of the historical record, to add to the understanding of the varied use of groups undertaken by this Hull House resident, and to use this knowledge to inform contemporary social work practice. Yarros merits a deserved, though long-delayed, recognition of her life and contribution, and she offers today's group workers inspiration for our practice.

REFERENCES

Addams, J. ([1910] 1961). *Twenty years at Hull House*. New York: The New American Library of World Literature, Inc.

Addams, J. ([1912] 1970). *A new conscience and an ancient evil*. New York: The Arno Press.

Bryan, M.L.M. and Davis, A.F. (Eds.) (1990). *100 years at Hull-House*. Bloomington, IN: Indiana University Press.

Bryan, M.L.M., Slote, N., De Angury, M. (Eds.) (1996). *The Jane Addams papers: A comprehensive guide*. Bloomington, IN: Indiana University Press.

Carson, M. (1990). *Settlement folk: Social thought and the American settlement movement, 1885-1930*. Chicago: The University of Chicago Press.

Chen, C.M. (1996). *"The sex side of life": Mary Ware Dennett's pioneering battle for birth control and sex education*. New York: The New Press.

Chesler, E. (1992). *Woman of valor: Margaret Sanger and the birth control movement in America*. New York: Simon and Schuster, Inc.

Clarke, C.W. (1961). *Taboo: The story of the pioneers of social hygiene*. Washington, DC: Public Affairs Press.

Costin, L. (1980). Edith Abbott. In B. Sicherman and C.H. Green (Eds.), *Notable American women: The modern period*. Cambridge, MA: Harvard University Press.

Davis, A.F. and McCree, M.L. (Eds.) (1969). *Eighty years at Hull-House*. Chicago: Quadrangle Books.

Ditzion, S. (1969). *Marriage, morals and sex in America: A history of ideas.* New York: W.W. Norton and Co., Inc.

Eaton, I. (1894). Hull-House and some of its distinctive features. *The Smith College Monthly,* 1(7), 1-10.

Gordon, L. (1977). *Woman's body, woman's right.* New York: Penguin Books.

Hamilton, A. (1910). Excessive child-bearing as a factor in infant mortality. *American Academy of Medicine,* 11(February), 181-187.

Hamilton, A. (1925). Poverty and birth control. *Birth Control Review,* August, 226-229.

Hamilton, A. ([1943] 1985). *Exploring the dangerous trades.* Boston: Little, Brown and Company.

Haslett, D.C. (2001). Yarros, Rachelle Slobodinsky. In R.L. Shultz and A. Hast, *Women building Chicago 1790-1990.* Bloomington, IN: Indiana University Press.

Holmes, R.W., Hamilton, A., Hedger, C., Bacon, C.S., and Stowe, H.M. (1908). The midwives of Chicago. *Journal of the American Medical Association,* April 25, 1346-1350.

Johnson, M.A. (Ed.) (1990). *The many faces of Hull House.* Chicago: University of Illinois Press.

Kelly, F. (1919). Quoted in At Social Worker's Convention. *Birth Control Review,* 3(7), 14.

Kennedy, D. (1970). *Birth control in America: The career of Margaret Sanger.* New Haven, CT: Yale University Press.

Lasch, C. (1971). Rachelle Slobodinsky Yarros. In E.T. Jones, J.W. James, and P.S. Boyer (Eds.), *Notable American women: 1607-1950.* Cambridge, MA: Harvard University Press.

Lee, P.R. (1937). *Social work as cause and function and other papers.* New York: Columbia University Press.

Lissak, R.S. (1989). *Pluralism and progressives: Hull House and the new immigrants, 1890-1919.* Chicago: University of Chicago Press.

Mackevich, E., Ruoff, G.W., and Vavra, L. (Eds.) (1989). *Opening new worlds: Jane Addams' Hull House.* Chicago: The University of Illinois at Chicago.

Polikoff, B.G. (1999). *With one bold act: The story of Jane Addams.* Chicago: Boswell Books.

Reed, J. (1978). *The birth control movement and American society.* Princeton, NJ: Princeton University Press.

Rosenblatt, R. and Waldfogel, D. (1983). *Handbook of clinical social work.* San Francisco, CA: Jossey-Bass Publishers.

Sanger, M. ([1938] 1971). *Margaret Sanger: An autobiography.* New York: Dover Publications, Inc.

Sicherman, B. (1984). *Alice Hamilton: A life in letters.* Cambridge, MA: Harvard University Press.

Stebner, E.J. (1997). *The women of Hull House: A study in spirituality, vocation, and friendship.* Albany, NY: State University of New York Press.

Ward, P.S. (1986). Yarros, Rachelle Slobodinsky. In Trattner, W.I., *Biographical dictionary of social welfare in America* (pp. 811-816). New York: Greenwood Press.

Ward, P.S. (1990). *At the eye of the storm: Hull House and the Chicago birth control debate.* A paper presented at Hull House and the People's Health: A Public Humanities Symposium, University of Illinois at Chicago, April 7.

Yarros, R.S. (1919a). Experiences of a lecturer. *Social Hygiene*, 5(2), 205-222.

Yarros, R.S. (1919b). Social Hygiene Committee report in the annual report of Women's City Club of Chicago. *Woman's City Club Bulletin*, Chicago, IL.

Yarros, R.S. (1920). Summary of the social hygiene work done from February 1, 1919 to June 1, 1920, under the auspices of the Division of Social Hygiene, Department of Public Health. *Woman's City Club Bulletin*, 5-9.

Yarros, R.S. (1925). Birth control and its relation to health and welfare. *The Medical Woman's Journal*, 268-272.

Yarros, R.S. (1929). Cost of medical care and the controversy with the Chicago Medical Society. *The Medical Woman's Journal*, 36, 261-264.

Yarros, R.S. (1931a). Objections disproved by clinical findings. *Birth Control Review*, 15(1), 15-16.

Yarros, R.S. (1931b). Sex education and pre-parental education. *Journal of Social Hygiene*, 17(9), 505-514.

Yarros, R.S. (1932a). The future of the birth control clinic. *Birth Control Review*, 26(11), 266-268.

Yarros, R.S. (1932b). Pre-marital, marital and parental consultation service. *The Medical Woman's Journal*, 32, 197-199.

Yarros, R.S. (1933). *Modern woman and sex: A feminist physician speaks.* Girard, KS: Haldeman-Julius Publications.

Yarros, R.S. (1938a). The national health conference. *The Medical Woman's Journal*, 45, 311-313.

Yarros, R.S. (1938b). *Sex problems in modern society.* Girard, KS: Haldeman-Julius Publications (republication).

Yarros, R.S. (1943). Women physicians and the problems of women. *The Medical Woman's Journal*, 43, 28-30.

Chapter 4

Social Group Work in Germany: An American Import and Its Historical Development

Jürgen Kalcher

INTRODUCTION

This chapter is conceived as a political chapter—as a chapter on democracy and on certain aspects of its practical implementation in a postwar situation. Its purpose is to document, to reflect, and to preserve some of the pragmatic outcomes of an American strategy on how to deal with a defeated enemy, whom they nevertheless regarded as human, in principle, and of worth to be educated or, rather, reeducated. This includes respect for the German culture and people, as acknowledged in history.

I attained a new understanding of the relevance of my subject when John Ramey wrote to the lecturers of this symposium eight days after the September 11 attack on the World Trade Center in New York City:

> These are unusual and tragic times. . . . Our democracy in the USA and the very idea of democracy are under attack. Thus it is important that we gather to maintain momentum and vigilance of democracy and freedom of association in societies everywhere. You'll find that idea as integral to the theme of the symposium.

This chapter is also meant as a contribution of solidarity with our attacked American friends, thus underlining what was supposed to be and has been the result of an American investment into democratization of our country after the war, through education of the German people (at least the Western portion of them), expecting them to walk on the humanistic and democratic side of the street along with all other members of democratic societies in the world, full of grief and deep sorrow over the many dead and wounded.

My chapter represents a rather subjective point of view. I'm predominantly talking about real-life experiences living during the first ten years of my life in a Nazi society, attending school, listening to the radio and to political discussions among the adults, being bombed, being evacuated, fleeing from the Soviet Red Army, living under Soviet occupation in the part that later became GDR, landing as a refugee in West Germany, and finally getting the chance to become and settle down as a citizen of a democratic society. I am also talking about the beginning of my professional career as a social group worker.

From the very platform of my life experience, I learned to understand intimately the high value of education in a historical situation that was marked by mutual feelings of revenge, of punishing the guilty, of hanging the responsible. That pattern had prevailed for thousands of years and had previously been applied by the Germans to their defeated enemies. In contrast with that ancient moral, the American principle was not to return evil with evil. However, that's easier said than done. You cannot accomplish high aspirations like that without having a strategy. Still, even then, putting it into action means to take a high risk because the concrete outcomes of such historical processes cannot really be predicted. They might go in the wrong direction. So, amazingly enough, it was trust in human nature that was at the onset of that educational endeavor. But could they trust people who had committed such terrible crimes as the Holocaust? Therefore, certain preconditions had to be provided. One of those preconditions was a roughly structured program, the American re-educational program for the defeated Germans.

REEDUCATING THE GERMAN PEOPLE

I cannot and do not want to approach the subject as a historian. If I did, I would have to discuss the causes of World War II, the American image of humans during the time of the New Deal under Franklin D. Roosevelt, and, last but not least, the American interpretation and philosophy of "democracy." A few historical facts have to be taken into account to understand the implications of that operation called "reeducation of the Germans," which means the elimination of all Nazi content and Nazi attitudes in a generation reared under Nazism, and to define instead "the broad principles governing the restoration of democratic political life to the country."[1]

Both aspects, however, are standing for different parts of what could be called a human engineering project. It seems indispensable to mark the difference between (1) getting rid of the Nazi ideology—the "cleansing"—and (2) replacing Nazi ideology by what we may call democratic values or just democracy. The first, labeled as *denazification,* followed the principle of destruction. It consisted in setting up a judicial and administrative system of punishing the culprits, of removing all Nazi content from public (and private) life by means of censoring schoolbooks or newspapers, prohibiting all Nazi symbols, restricting the freedom of assembly, etc. The second aspect however was the one that promised true efficiency. The new method, the real new way to handle the problem, contained the very essence of reeducation, namely, to educate the former enemy in the spirit and towards the goals of democracy. This approach aimed to build up and develop a new system.

The concept of reeducating a whole people had been born during the war at about 1943, or even earlier. British as well as American high-ranking politicians and military personnel made suggestions as to how to change the norms of the German society, and by that change the Germans themselves. The image of "a German" was at that time—how could it be different?—mainly determined by the bogeyman image of a cruel enemy. Therefore, there were not only high humanistic intentions that motivated the large program but, let's say, a mixture of hatred, arrogance, naivety, and an enormous portion of helplessness. However, among all that you may also discover that humanistic, positive kernel or core. Somehow that cruel breed consisted of human beings, and human beings—this was their conviction—could be changed by educating them or, in other terms, by making them learn.

Another consideration was that there existed different types of perpetrators, namely, real criminals who could not be changed and had to be punished and others who were just fellow travelers of the Nazi party, who were able to learn and to profit from an educational program in a democratic sense. So it seemed to be necessary to find out who was who and then submit them to different treatments. A means to do this task of assessment was the method of "screening." By means of questionnaires the probationers were put into different categories.

Reeducation actually started in some of the British and American camps for POWs (as they were called) at a time when the war was reaching its peak. Camp 300 and Wiston House were examples of British camps. The Factory at Fort Kearney and the important center at Eustis as well as camps at Getty and Wetherhill were examples of the American endeavor to "produce" democratic Germans, who were determined to be the seed of a new beginning in their home country as soon as the war ended.[2]

I know from a very good friend of mine, who was twenty-one when he became a POW in England, that he was offered academic courses and that those courses were very well organized and well done. He still shows proudly the many notes he took in a course of clinical psychology and psychoanalysis. He later became a psychologist and psychotherapist.

We have to be aware, however, that making the "Huns" learn the right things, that instructing, informing, and teaching a selected group of war prisoners, was quite another matter compared to reeducating the whole people. Although the same basic principles were applied, this postwar educational enterprise was by far much more complicated ad problematic than the former. As an important document I would recommend the authentic novel by Ernst von Salomon, *The Questionnaire,*[3] showing the problems and pitfalls of that bureaucratic instrument and its impact on the reality of life. It also shows the impossibility of being able to overturn the whole structure of a criminal political system.

As a matter of fact, most historians and also the majority of the average German contemporaries agreed on the failure of those restrictive measures.[4] As one of the critical commentators formulates, "However, the way in which denazification developed over time not only made a mockery of justice but also, in the end, defeated any broader educational purposes,"[5] and the author argues in detail that there were no set criteria as to who qualified as a bona fide Nazi and who did not, and into which of the four "guilty" categories people should be assigned. Then there was no clear consent among those who occupied Germany. The Americans "sternly believed in separating the guilty from the innocent," the British—very formal—tried the same but even more stringent, punishing the ones who were "formally guilty" and on the other hand missing many of the real culprits. Whereas the Soviets "exculpated the Nazis in their own Zone . . . opening them the ranks of their . . . Communist institutions," the French on their part believed in Nazism as an "endemic quality of the German Volk" being incapable of reconstruction, so they "concentrated only on the worst offenders in their Zone, trying them swiftly and expeditiously." Also, with the onset of the cold war, Washington sought Germany's support and was even more ready to forgive and forget, happily backed by capitalist right-wingers at home. Thus, as the author concludes, the denazification ended up in some kind of renazification because "the renewed rise of radical movements on the right after 1945 turned out to be partly the result of Allied policy."

Also this author cites an observer of Germany saying that "democracy to Germans meant simply 'carbonated soft drinks like Coca-Cola, chewing gum, baseball and anti-Communism'."

From my point of view this is a rather authentic description of the political situation at about 1950. Many people I knew at that time seemed to be disillusioned, apolitical, very egocentric, and often cynical. The result was an overall attitude of "without me . . . "; the Germans even spoke of an *Ohne-mich-Bewegung* (Without-Me-Movement), calling individual persons an *Ohnemichel* (Without-Me-Michael). There is no denying the fact, however, that there were also others who were beginning to question the old national socialistic truths and opening up to a new beginning.

What really failed was—as Kater calls it—the "political reconditioning of a people." To put it into behavioral therapeutic terms, negative conditioning always needs to be supported by some positive additions or gains, and there was too much negative conditioning (destruction) in that experiment and too little of a positive perspective. If you take anything away from the client, the purpose of therapy will be missed. To give the Germans Coca-Cola and Hollywood and a fiction called democracy did not work. This holds especially true for that macro social experiment called denazification.

Why do I actually elaborate those old stories? First, I think the actual political world situation of 2001 is not so very much different from that in the mid-1940s, at least concerning how democratic structures and democratic values can be introduced into fundamentally authoritarian systems. Also, the situation of our East German compatriots after the fall of the Communist wall in 1998 includes many similar elements to the 1945 postwar situation. Other similar questions, for example, arise also when we look to former Yugoslavia or to Iraq or to Palestine, and even to Northern Ireland. Or—and this seems to be extremely relevant to the present—when we ask ourselves what has to be done in Afghanistan as soon as the political power has been taken over by Western democratic systems or at least is governed under Western influence.

The other reason—and that is the main reason in our context—for going back into the history of World War II is to show how some daring humanists, whom I call peace bringers, were able to successfully and convincingly influence and shape a new democratic generation in my country, and that this had and has to do with social work with groups. And you will understand why I call social group work an American import. It's only if we understand some of the complex and awkward preconditions that we may estimate the work of certain individuals who had an approach other than the one of the official military administration.

A DIFFERENT APPROACH:
EDUCATIONAL PROCESSES TARGETING
GERMAN YOUTH

Interaction (Interdependence)

> Kater writes: As a consequence of a collapsed political culture, the need of reeducation, broadly conceived to incorporate both the political and the intellectual sectors, remained paramount from the mid-1940s to the mid-1960s. While the older generation posed formidable problems of resentment (recalcitrance), suspicion and apathy, German youth was a more promising source of concentration.[6]

Compared to those authoritarian methods of manipulation, we should keep in mind that reeducation, as all education, is a process of interaction, which means that there are always two sides of the coin. If there are on one side individuals full of resistance against taking over a new political culture from their war enemies, there are on the other hand the methods of education they are going to apply. Those methods that failed were abstract, bureaucratic instruments popped on them by a military administration. They had a chance to be successful only if they were connected with real personal engagement.[7] One of the mistakes the Allied Forces made in implementing their ideas of reeducation was that they neglected the interdependence of such processes and did not even pay attention to the very nature of education as a broad process instead of just instruction or even preaching. That means keeping in mind that the intended changes would take a lot of time and would principally be open in regard to the ends.

Peacemakers

The decision of the Allies at the Potsdam Conference in July 1945 to assist in the reeducation of a German generation reared under Nazism raised not only those ethical and methodological questions but also the question of who should do that job, and, last but not least, the question of the costs. No need to mention that there existed severe problems of different political currents. There was rivalry and competition, for instance, between the New Dealers around FDR and his Secretary of the Treasury, Hans Morgenthau, and their liberal opponents, and also the leftists, who pursued their special political goals. They all, however, agreed "that the United States should follow its democratic mission in the world."[8]

Another relevant problem concerned the recruiting of government officials to be engaged in the democratization policies. Most of them were intellectuals, linguists, political scientists, psychologists, educators, and, as we know, social workers, some of whom were social group workers. Mostly, the German specialists were of German heritage, either immigrants or Germans in exile, as, for example, Thomas Mann, who became one of the members of the U.S. Committee for the Reeducation of National Socialist Prisoners of War in 1944.

Examples

Taking all this as background information, the special story of using social work, and within that social group work, as a method of democratizing and reeducating the Germans started somewhere in the first years after the war. I mentioned earlier "peace bringers," and I would now like to give a few examples of what and whom I mean.

As I know from Gisela Konopka there were individual persons and committees traveling through Germany in the late 1940s and early 1950s in order to understand, in particular, the situation of the German youth and to find points of departure for democratic education. Politically it was clear then, that further development of the European states would not work without a functioning German democracy. So the youth needed to be the focus. Therefore, points of interest were, in the first place, schools and universities and then the educational system in general. Also, youth centers were founded in the American and the British Zone (later BI-Zone), offering all kinds of political and educational courses and workshops.

Another reason for developing such activities was the deep need and poverty and the deep decline of that postwar generation in Germany. Millions of people who had lost their roots in their home provinces in the East, now occupied by the Red Army, had lost relatives and many had also lost their health. Destroyed cities and devastated factories and industries not only formed a dangerous potential for future peace in Europe and in the world but were also the subject of humanistic considerations, touching the hearts of many a member of Western societies. So a broad wave of supports and signs of sympathy with the former enemy rolled over the Western Zones of Germany. As an example, let me mention the CARE movement that brought considerable relief for many suffering families (and functioned as an example and encouragement for many people in Germany to later on—and still today—support suffering people all over the world by sending them packages and all kinds of goods besides the official payments).

Among those travelers on behalf of humanity was also an English publisher, Victor Gollancz, who had lost many of his Jewish relatives and friends in the Holocaust. He was one of the first who brought the situation in Germany to the attention of his compatriots by writing a book, *In Darkest Germany,* and as the speaker of the relief organization Save Europe Now, he appealed compassionately to the public to prevent children and youth in Germany from becoming sadly neglected and morally dissolute. Somewhat later a foundation was named after him, sponsoring especially young social workers or students in this field. I myself had the privilege of becoming a Gollancz scholar. Later Victor Gollancz was highly honored in the German Bundesrepublik on behalf of his outstanding services to protect the welfare of the postwar generation in Germany.

Others were sent to Germany as social workers—and I am concentrating on only the social work sector, leaving out other areas, such as economy, science, industry, etc. Among them were Henry B. Ollendorff from Cleveland; Gisela Konopka from Minneapolis; Ruby Pernell, also from Cleveland; Kurt Reichert, now in San Diego; or Magda Kelber, returning from emigration in England—just to mention some of them, because they were group workers. Others, like Anne Fischer from Richmond, shaped a whole new generation of German social work students by introducing the principles of social casework into the philosophy of the German social welfare system.

Magda Kelber along with Christa von Schenck became the founders of Haus Schwalbach near Frankfurt. For many years Haus Schwalbach was the very center of social group work in Western Germany, editing the journal *Schwalbacher Blätter* and teaching courses for social workers, educators, or teachers. Although they did not apply the notion social group work, but called it *Gruppenpädagogik,* thus picking up, or rather adding to, the old struggle in the United States.[9] They made a very important contribution towards democratization of social services. Here I'm only pointing out the very first ambassadors and do not mention in detail such important theorists as Louis Lowy and Hans S. Falck, whose influence on social group work in Germany, at a later date, was tremendous.

My very special reverence is directed to Henry B. Ollendorff,[10] who also started out as a group work instructor in Germany. As the holder of a doctorate in law from the University of Heidelberg he had left Germany because of being severely hindered in his juridical work, in particular by the racial discrimination laws. After thirteen months of solitary confinement, he was finally acquitted of the charge and emigrated to the United States in 1938. He and his wife became American citizens. Henry Ollendorff studied a second time, this time social work in New York, and started to work with Cleveland's underprivileged children.

In 1954 the U.S. Department of State asked Ollendorff to go to Germany to work for their reeducational program. He started out conducting courses for youth leaders and social workers at Haus Schwalbach for five months. But his experiences with those young people motivated him to start his own program, bringing those people to the States for about half a year. There he provided for housing with Cleveland families, taking an introductory course at Western Reserve, and working in different field assignments under the same conditions as their American colleagues.

Ollendorff's motivation, as remembered by his wife, Martha, seems to me to be typical for the majority of the mostly Jewish social work ambassadors to Germany:

> My life was saved. I want to dedicate my life to assuring that something like the Holocaust never happens again. People, especially youth, must learn early to respect religious, racial or other differences, understand each other and to live together.

Thus, in 1956, he went to his former homeland where he and his family had been persecuted, bringing with him twenty-five German youth leaders and social workers, whom he thought to be "multipliers," to live with Cleveland families and attend Western Reserve, where he, along with other teachers—among them Margaret Hartford and Grace L. Coyle—introduced the foreign students to American social work in theory and practice. No need to mention that within twenty-five years his program extended enormously. Almost all the states in the world were sending their participants to the United States, and about fourteen American university cities participated as hosts in the name of the American way of life. Later on they sent their own students to those countries, since in 1960 former participants founded a reverse program (CIF—Cleveland International Fellowship), inviting professionals from abroad to their own countries, preserving and maintaining also the "spirit of Henry"—the basic humanistic roots of democracy. The purposes of CIF were officially formulated as "[p]romotion of education, elementary and vocational training including student help, and [p]romotion of international ways of thinking, tolerance towards all fields of culture and the idea of international understanding." In the pursuit of this, they often sponsor biennial conferences around the world.

Not going too much into the details of the CIP/CIF history (changed from Cleveland International Program for Youthleaders and Social Workers to Council of International Programs . . .), I want to describe the enormous snowball effect it had in the name of peace and humanity.

As I myself got the opportunity to participate in CIP in 1960, which brought me to Cleveland, Ohio, and to Camp Wediko (therapeutic summer camp for emotionally disturbed boys run by the Boston Judge Baker Child Guidance Center in the New Hampshire woods), I experienced very intimately the consequences for my future. Back in Hamburg I started a degree in psychology, thus trying to fill the gap in knowledge of which I had become aware during my participation in CIP.

It was another Jewish emigrant returning home from the United States who, without his knowledge, motivated me to choose the university of Hamburg to become a psychologist: Curt Bondy, a former assistant professor at the William Stern Psychological Institute in Hamburg before 1933.[11] Curt Bondy had returned to Hamburg in 1950, when he had been asked to take over the former William Stern Chair in Psychology, bringing along with him a substantial sum of money for building up psychology in Germany as well as new methods and theories. His first project was the standardization of the Wechsler Intelligence Scales for children and for adults, by this marking the beginning of a new era in psychology. Another pioneering innovation he introduced was the classical child guidance approach. As the holder of this academic chair, he was the only university teacher in (Western) Germany who, besides psychology, represented, taught, and helped to develop social work within a university teaching program.

What I did not know at that time, and only realized in 1994 when I met Gisela Konopka, was that he not only knew Gisela but had cooperated with her and Henry B. Ollendorff in CIP.

Actually, many other names should be added. It is a long list of individuals who had been driven out of their homes because they were Jewish—as the great majority of them—or had belonged to a socialist or other political party or organization were oppositional to the NSDAP (National Socialist German Workers' Party, as their full name was) and their regime.

It is not possible to list them all. However, much of this memorizing work has been done in the last years in my country, as, for example, in the book by Joachim Wieler and Susanne Zeller, *Emigrierte Sozialarbeit—Portraits vertriebener SoziarbeiterInnen,* from 1995.[12] So let me instead take one example for all: Gisela Konopka.

ONE FOR ALL: GISELA KONOPKA

I would like to start this section by quoting what she wrote when I asked her in 1994 to write a foreword for an evaluative booklet on the Hansische Jugendbund (HJB), a Hamburg group work project that was started in 1947 by Elisabeth Sülau, and which stopped in 1967. It had been supported by, among others, Gisela Konopka in a twofold way: indirectly, by handing over, or rather translating, group work philosophy and methodology into the German postwar social welfare system (especially youth welfare), and directly, by teaching and advising the HJB workers during several stays in Germany. What is significant for her motivations and her attitude towards Germany seems to be best illustrated by her own words:[13]

Elisabeth Sülau—what great memories!

I had returned to Germany in 1950 and 1951 to help with the restoration of youth services, children institutions, and to work with delinquent young people after the destructive period of the Nazis. The American government had asked me to do this and I accepted. Many of my friends chided me for going back to help those who had demeaned me because I am Jewish, who had killed almost all my relatives, who had put me in a concentration camp because of my anti-Nazi activities, and had taken away my German nationality and made me "stateless."

I had seen the terror of the Nazis in Austria, in France, and had finally arrived penniless in the United States. I was reunited with my husband, who had also been an anti-Nazi fighter, and a new life had started in the United States.

I was teaching Social Group Work at the University. It had much meaning to me because its philosophy was based on the understanding that all human beings are interdependent and that in working with people and especially with children and youth, one had to help them to be strong and caring individuals. The individual is important and so is the group. "Gemeinschaft" must not suffocate the individual, and the individual needs the support of the group and community and can contribute to it. Such a concept of "group work" could help to restore humanities to youth services.

I also went back to Germany because I felt that one must not punish the children for the sins of their elders.

And then there was Hamburg, the place where I had been in the Gestapo cellar, but also the place where I had worked with others, Jews and non-Jews, against the Nazis. I met Elisabeth Sülau and we felt like sisters. She understood that one must accept everybody as a human being regardless of who they are, how they look, what race, religion, etc. She accepted the prostitutes and the pimps and let them learn how life can be different without exploiting others or allowing oneself to be exploited.

And she ends regarding the continuing group work after that time of the HJB:

[T]his work is based on the premise that the human being is not a "thing" to be pushed around or made into someone's image, but is a significant individual who can develop and respect others with their differences and similarities as human beings.

This text sounds very familiar to our contemporary perception—nothing new, we may say. Looking back, however, to the year 1950 and understanding the background on which Gisela's and the others' peace work began, we may realize the incredible gap between Nazi ideology and the new message. So Gisela Konopka, when coming to the United States in the late 1930s, expressed her own fascination of that philosophy of social group work:[14]

For myself . . . I must say that my first encounter with social group work in 1941 was a revelation. Having just come from a society that seemed to present an inescapable gulf between the individual and the group—which insisted that the individual be sacrificed to the interests of the group—I found the concept of individualization in and through the group exhilarating.

Yet Gisela was very much aware of the other side of groups, the dangerous potentials they also contain:

On the other hand, [groups] also told the story of the disastrous power of group associations and of the skilled misuse that could be made of them. It taught group workers, who at times had considered group activities a value in themselves, that these activities, too, could be used to enslave youth as well as to help them freely participate in a human society.

Whenever I read these statements I see before my eyes—and sometimes in reality, because it is still there—the memorial for the many German soldiers who had been killed in World Wars I and II. Soldiers are depicted marching around a large stone block in their uniforms, and the inscription reads, "Deutschland must live, even when we are bound to die." This to me signifies the enormous challenge of the new democratic values and attitudes and structures, which were imported to my country by individual peace bringers, as in opposition to Hitler's image of the German youth as being "hard as Krupp steel, tough like leather and as fast as greyhounds." As the Hitlerjugend used to sing, "Our flag means more than our death."

THE HANSISCHE JUGENDBUND—
A DEMOCRATIC GROUP WORK AGENCY

St. Pauli is a red-light area in Hamburg with a long tradition. Alcohol and prostitution close by the harbor were characteristic and substantial features of that part of the city. When I started the second half year of my internship between the school of social work and entering the profession in 1959, HJB had just moved to this place. This was the forth residence of that unique place for children and youth since its foundation in 1947. In the 1960s they became the neighbors of the place where a new unknown band from Liverpool was plying their own songs: The Beatles.

Elisabeth Sülau had started that work as a meeting point for young folks under supervision of the Hamburg Youth Authorities, and in the first time they were meeting in the living room of Mrs. Sülau, who was then a youth care worker in Hamburg. Before the war she had been an active member of the Freideutsche Jugend, an association belonging to the Jugendbewegung (youth movement before World War I and between the wars consisting of a cluster of different groups and organizations representing all kinds of political, religious, or ideological youth activities). This movement had been silently taken over by the Hitlerjugend since 1933. Gisela Konopka herself had been a member of one of those youth associations, like many active and innovative young middle-class people of both sexes. There had also been a similar movement in the working class—wandering out of the gray walls of the industrial cities; living a modest life out in the countryside; being honest and open, clear and pure; living their lives as self-determined youth; doing all they wanted to do in a group; neglecting the old authorities, ready to set out for a new future. These were some of their central ideals. You may understand that these values were highly appreciated by the national socialists. Many of the young folks—not all of them—were pure idealists and refused to be political, so they did not become aware of the political intentions of the Nazis. But, as soon as they became aware that they had gone in the wrong direction, they were already captured by the Nazis and involved in Nazi activities.

After World War II, German youth workers, teachers, and other people, who took over responsibility for that postwar youth, started to look for historical threads they could use to establish a new cultural basis for raising and educating a new democratic generation. By separating the means from the political goals, they presented and represented those new values but took over the idealism and the means of the pre-Nazi Jugendbewegung. So living in the peer group, hiking in the countryside, cooking on an open campfire, and singing the old songs were preserved. In the eyes of the majority of the German democrats of that time they were not suspect. Most people regarded them as being some kind of scouts' group. They were seen as one of the very few connections to history that seemed to be free from national socialist ideology. The new democratic values were soaked up and were seen as an enrichment and innovation in youth life.

What was new in Sülau's approach was to extend this kind of youth life even to those young folks who were social dropouts or marginal or even juvenile delinquents. The Hansische Jugendbund opened up for those youth who before had been restricted, isolated, and persecuted by state officials, and not only for political reasons. From the beginning, and particularly in the 1950s, her group work approach was supported by books and papers on social group work as a method of social work, and especially by personal advice, workshops, lectures, etc., held by Curt Bondy and Gisela Konopka. Indirectly, there was another influence on her work, namely, the many social work students who spent their internships in the HJB, bringing in new theoretical knowledge from their schools, which vice versa were also influenced by American book translations and teachers from the United States, as I described earlier.

It would be another lecture, though, to describe in detail what that work over twenty years really was like. In 1967, when Elisabeth Sülau, whom all the members called "Ambrosius" (actually as an expression of an antiauthoritarian attitude), retired, this work could no longer be sustained. But the democratic spirit was carried over into other organizational forms. Social group work in Hamburg was reorganized and continued in a new organizational structure by Lisel Werninger up until the 1980s.

Eighteen years after the decline of the HJB, in 1985, some former members of the HJB—then in their forties or even their midfifties—remembered those "good times" and decided to take a boat trip on the Elbe River. Doubts about whether it would be possible to reach a substantial crowd of people turned out to be irrelevant. More than 150 former juvenile members showed up, thanks to word-of-mouth propaganda, and had a wonderful time. There was a mixture of all classes, professions, and ages—all returning home in high spirits.

Shortly after this event Christel Gasterstaedt, a former staff member and close friend of Elisabeth Sülau, invited many of the participants to be interviewed by her, trying to find out about the efficiency of that early social group work in HJB, which was really fundamental political education and preparation for a democratic lifestyle.

Evaluating the HJB Approach

Some of the results, as summarized in the book I mentioned,[15] are the following. When a former member, in looking back to her experiences in the HJB, points out that "self organizing of the group was something I probably liked best, because I had to take over responsibility," this shows in essence what the majority of the members felt. From the beginning they had developed democratic structures like statutes, a parliament, a court, a newspaper, etc. Within this frame of reference, much of the participation of the young people could be realized, and it amazed me, when I started my work in 1959 in the club, how self-confident those youngsters were. When I realized that many of them had been very problematic youth, I was even more impressed.

There was the big open group, where all kinds of young people from the neighborhood as well as from other parts of the city were welcome and encouraged to join different activities, and there were the small face-to-face-groups, for which the young folks were selected and invited to become members. The group process was planned for about two to three years. There were some groups of special interests, but most of them were "friendship groups," as they were called. It was part of the group structure that there were always two leaders: the professional group worker and one of the group members, to be elected by the group. The social group worker was called *Gruppenberater* (group adviser) and the appointed group member was called *Gruppenleiter* (group leader). You may imagine that this construct was not easy to manage (I hate this expression in this connection!), but it was one of the most efficient means of participation of the young group members, since it was invested with real power.

One of the former group leaders remembered:

> In 1952 I was elected group leader of the "City Club." I had to attend the group leader meetings and had to organize weekend trips for the whole group. I was also elected member of parliament and became even provisional chairman for half a year. . . . As the chairman I had to act for the HJB in the public and had to deal with states officers of the Hamburg Youth Authorities— Me, who hated these officers. In the company, where I was trained to become a commercial clerk, I was elected youth representative, later I became a trade union member. I was able to be politically active, because I had learned in the HJB to make and keep the records and not to be afraid to say my opinion in public.

No need to underline that these were new fields to be tilled, and that it was strange to many of the officials that the ones who accomplished these tasks were (former) clients. Therefore, there was much distrust and ill will on the part of the public authorities, especially as they had to pay for it.

Although those groups were not conceived as (psycho)therapeutic groups, there were many statements made as to report fundamental personality changes and lasting gains. For instance, an over-fifty-year-old lady reported:

The group gave me a lot of security. At that time I was very shy, reserved and unsociable, particularly as far as boys were concerned. On our flight in 1944 I had been raped by a Russian soldier and therefore I didn't want to dance with boys. But little by little I gained confidence in the group. All the group members supported me not to run away from boys.

Another told about his personal development:

A social worker made the proposal to send me to the HJB. Before my mother had brought me into sort of detention home. I begged her to take me home again. I was always fighting with my mother. She treated me unfairly. She was never content with my achievements at school and when she thought she could no longer cope with me she called up my uncle, who gave me an awful thrashing. Our relatives called me a "boaster." Coming to the HJB I felt like shit at first. I brought some classmates and we founded our own group "Die Sturmvogel" ("Birds of the Storm"). I believe I have been very much molded through my group experiences in the Club. What I needed then was love and acknowledgement. And I got it there. There it was possible to settle conflicts and disharmonies within a family atmosphere.

All and many more of these reports and narratives can be found in the booklet I mentioned. Taken all together, it is estimated that about 5,000 individuals, in the course of the existence of the HJB, had been members and had been touched and shaped to a certain degree by their group experiences in this unique piece of youth work. They developed an understanding of democratic values and attitudes and became "multipliers" in the German postwar society.

BY WAY OF SUMMARY

There had been a terrible war between 1939 and 1945 in Europe. Hitler and Germany had been defeated and destroyed. One of the purposes for the United States to go into this war had been for the sake of democracy. One of the urgent questions after the war was how to deal with the defeated enemy. As far as I can see, this was the first time in history that the victory was not, in the first place, used to hang the culprits and, then, to exploit the losers, but to educate the whole German people in the name of democracy. In this way serious mistakes were made, and to some degree the whole action called reeducation was a failure; certainly denazification can be seen as a failure.

On the other side there were certain personalities, humanistic peace bringers, who believed in the very power of democracy and humanistic values. As messengers of a new political beginning, they used the reeducational program in a different way—in the name of humanity. Their personal venture and dedication was convincing, especially as a great number among them were Jews who had lost their relatives in the Holocaust and who had suffered the loss of their homes and their property. To go back to Germany with the best of intentions, giving back with full hands, is an almost unbelievable innovation in the historical line. An ethical attitude for them was more important than material gains. In spite of an uncertain outcome, they took the risk and the responsibility for their endeavors. Social workers played an essential part—it is their merit that Germany developed a strong democratic system in terms of policy, economy, and culture. They were human beings who had grown with their pains but who were also pragmatists who hoped to implement their high aspirations.

I think that the time has come not only to write down this part of postwar history that has to do with social group work but also to say thank you. The American belief in democratic values has long since also become a high value in Germany, and there are many examples to support bringing it to other people. Today it is our feeling of solidarity, following the attack on democracy on September 11, 2001, which is shared by the large majority of the Germans, East and West, that I also want to convey. That Germany today is one of the most reliable partners of the United States and of their democratic friends is due to the women and men who decided not to return evil with evil. As Henry Ollendorff used to say, one man can make a difference. But stop! Does not this hold true also for Hitler and Stalin? Therefore, we have to think further.

John Ramey, by reminding us of momentum and vigilance, makes us also reflect on our own part in that deadly play of today. What could possibly be the insult given to cause people of other cultures and beliefs to attack the very heart of capitalism? Wasn't the World Trade Center the symbol of the abstract, impersonal, and uncanny power of money—the god of our globalized world?

Also, will bombing be the only and adequate answer, setting off destruction with destruction, evil by evil? As long as the true reasons for that disgusting act are not understood, bombing will bear a high risk of inflaming the whole Arabic and Moslem part of the world; some are already speaking of a struggle of cultures. We ought to reflect also on the damaging side effects on some of our own citizens, looking for a chance to prove their own Ramboism, and on what will happen when we are declaring the war on terrorism. And should not that war on poverty be continued along with a new understanding of the roots of terrorism?

Let me, dear friends, just raise the questions. I do not know the answers in a down-to-earth sense. But I learned from those peace bringers, whom I mentioned before, that revenge cannot be the only and general answer. I learned also from their engagement that an adequate reaction has to include direct, personal commitment and has to respect the long duration of processes leading to peace in the world. Let me quote again what Henry Ollendorff once said: "The Americans always produced in their history the power of innovation—thus being able to overcome whatever the challenge might have been."

Let me end with these, maybe critical, thoughts, standing on the grounds of democracy and of a real friendship between our nations:

> Monarchy is like a splendid ship, with all sails set; it moves majestically on, then it hits a rock and sinks forever. Democracy is like a raft. It never sinks, but damn it, your feet are always in the water.[16]

NOTES

1. *An Outline of American History—The New Deal and World War.* Stockholm, Sweden: U.S. Information Agency, May 1994.

2. In detail, see Arnold Krammer, *Nazi Prisoners of War in America.* New York: Stein and Day Publishers, 1994.

3. Von Salomon, *Der Fragebogen* [The questionary]. Reinbek bei Hamburg: dtv, 1951.

4. See, for example, Clemens Vollnhals, *Entnazifizierung* [Denazification]. Reinbek bei Hamburg: dtv, 1991.

5. Michael H. Kater, *Problems of Political Reeducation in West Germany, 1945-1960.* Los Angeles: Simon Wiesenthal Center, Annual 4, 1997; see pp. 2-3.

6. Ibid., p. 5.

7. There are good examples for this in Krammer, *Nazi Prisoners of War in America.*

8. Felicitas Hentschke, "Speak your mind even if your voice shakes!" Personal paper, February 19, 2000.

9. Compare Gisela Konopka, *Social Group Work: A Helping Process.* Englewood Cliffs, NJ: Prentice-Hall, 1963, pp. 9-11: "Kilpatrick thought that group work should be identified with the profession of education" (p. 11).

10. I'm following here G. Schmidt and G. Senssfelder, *Short Survey of the History of Cleveland International Fellowship in Germany.* Berlin: CIF-Germany (ed.), 2001.

11. Karl Gerlicher and Klaus Eyferth (eds.), *Erinnerungen an Curt Bondy anläblich seines 100 Geburtstages (1994)* [In memory of Curt Bondy on the occasion of his 100th birthday (1994)]. Erlangen: FIM-Psychologie, 1995.

12. Joachim Wieler and Susanne Zeller (eds.), *Emigrierte Sozialarbeit* [Social work emigrated]. Freiburg: Lambertus, 1995.

13. Christel Gasterstaedt (ed.), *Drauβen war Druck, aber im JHB konntest Du aufatmen* [Outside was stress, but in the HJB you could breathe again]. Hamburg, 1995, foreword, pp. 11-12; translation from the German.

14. Konopka, *Social Group Work*, p. 8.

15. See Gasterstaedt, *Drauβen war Druck.* All citations in this evaluation quoting former members of the NJB are translated into English from the chapter by Gerd Krüger, pp. 55-84.

16. D.W. Brogan, *The Free State.* London: Hamish Hamilton, 1944.

PART II:
CONTEMPORARY
APPLIED GROUP WORK

Chapter 5

Conflict As an Expression of Difference: A Desirable Group Dynamic in Anti-Oppression Social Work Practice

Nancy Sullivan

INTRODUCTION

Growth and development in our diverse contemporary community mean learning and enhancing interpersonal relationship skills and acquiring mutually accepting and affirming attitudes about and with other people. In an environment where "difference" is an integral reality and can present itself in social interrelating as conflict (that is, oppositional or antagonistic action), social group work may be an apt means to provide members with an opportunity for such learning in a dramatic, experiential way. This use of group work in social work practice relates to its early purposes of teaching responsible paths for personal growth and ongoing social and developmental change. Not initially for remediation or particular problem solving, social group work was seen as a means of supplementing, augmenting, or reinforcing the "normal" socialization process provided by families, and required by all people to equip them with social competencies for harmonious and effective living (Wilson and Ryland, 1949/1981; Kaiser, 1958/1980; Coyle, 1959/1980; Somers, 1962; Klein, 1970; Goroff, 1972).

This chapter addresses the functional concept of conflict in social group work, regarding it as a desirable, though challenging, dynamic in group life, and occurring as "an expression of difference." Acknowledging the current relevance and application of the foundation principles of our social group work heritage, it illustrates the facility of group process in a social work group as a context in which expression of difference may arise naturally, and as a means by which dealing with difference positively may be experienced and achieved.

The chapter attempts, as well, to link to present practice social group work's early purposes of preparing people with skills to enable them to participate in and ongoingly shape the very nature of society. Although the term *empowerment* did not appear regularly in our literature until the 1980s (for example, Hirayama and Hirayama, 1986), the concept has characterized the approach and goals of social group work practice throughout its history. Dealing with conflict as an expression of difference fits well with the anti-oppression approach to social work, which is increasingly prevalent in social work education and practice, the objectives of which include creating opportunities for marginalized people (those different from mainstream culture) to become, and be recognized as, full members of society. The ideological theme of respect runs concurrently through anti-oppression social work and through our social group work tradition. Applying respectful people-affirming values to deal with difference arising in a group reflects the early purposes of social group work, and may be a key factor in reframing conflict as a desirable group dynamic that serves as an opportunity to enable people to understand, appreciate, and be mutually and collectively enriched by "difference."

The following section lists ten principles for desirable conflict in social group work practice. The final section of the paper presents four vignettes of group life, with accompanying commentary to illustrate the principles evident in them.

PRINCIPLES FOR DESIRABLE CONFLICT

1. Conflict as an expression of difference may be welcomed, though initially dreaded. It signifies a willingness on the part of members to disagree openly or to expose their attitudes and understandings even when such expression provokes anger or discomfort in other members. Contrary to the fears of group workers, conflict is not an end or *the* end of a group. Bernstein (1978, p. 75) writes, "Conflict, often unpleasant and even nasty, is not a final end: . . . it is pervasive . . . in groups and . . . it has tremendous constructive possibilities if utilized skilfully and thoughtfully." Similarly reiterated in more recent times, Steinberg (1997, p. 161) sees conflict producing "a highly constructive state of affairs when it propels people to greater heights of

insight and sensitivity." An incident of conflict arising in a group can be an opportunity in the live, communal action to have one's previously held assumptions about "others" questioned and modified. This opportunity places the purposes of contemporary social group work within the framework of the historical vision and concept of the group as a vehicle of socialization.

2. Conflict must be acknowledged in the group as a critical focus of the moment. The emotional aspect of conflict may touch nerves in the various members, which may result in those members being unable to participate fully in the ongoing process due to their preoccupation with feelings such as anger, frustration, and hurt. "Conflict may diminish or go underground, but seldom goes away" (Coser, 1956, in Mondros, Woodrow, and Weinstein, 1992, p. 45). With courage, confidence, respect, and group work skills, the worker involves the group in exploring the issues of the conflict and acceptable resolution of it, for the continued maintenance of the group and service to individual members.

3. Conflict is full of meaning and usefulness in a group's life. It is a complex interrelational phenomenon with cognitive and affective components, embodied in social exchange. It can destroy a group, with members deciding it is too much pain or stress to attend, or it can be a vehicle, as "an integrative force in the group" (Simmel, 1955, p. 17), to help move the group towards a greater sense of wholeness, and to help advance the social development of individual members. A key factor in its effect on the group may be the skills of the worker. Intervening in conflict requires the worker to think and act in many ways simultaneously: to self-monitor one's own views on the issue; to mediate an active disagreement by attending to each party in terms of creating an opportunity for feelings and opinions to be expressed and clarified; and to assist the group as a whole to examine the differences and commonalities present among the members here and in the wider context of society, towards acceptable resolution.

4. Acceptable conflict resolution in the group may be expedited by worker intervention that first acknowledges that a difference has been expressed, and by presenting it as a difference in outlook, views, or understanding, rather than personalized as "Ralph says . . . , but Tom disagrees . . ." By depersonalizing or "disembodying" the difference, the whole group can be drawn into the exploration of the issue, lessening the possibility that specific individuals are labeled as right or

wrong, good or bad. The focus of discussion or debate becomes more generalized and conceptualized, a safer and potentially more productive forum to process the thorny content using the collective resources of the full membership. "True and effective conflict resolution" (Kurland and Salmon, 1998, p. 89) is achieved through "integration." Considered the ideal way of resolving conflict in groups, preferable to "domination" and even to "compromise," integration is a means by which "a new solution is reached and respected that includes the views of all 'sides'" (Kurland and Salmon, 1998, p. 89). Our literature holds a longtime historical account of references on integration as the most advantageous means and outcome of conflict resolution (Eubank, 1932, in Wilson and Ryland, 1949/1981, and in Bernstein, 1978; Follett, 1942, in Wilson and Ryland, 1949/1981).

5. Exploration of the issue begins with providing an opportunity for the perceived "offender" to clarify his or her meaning, and to explain the basis for the position expressed. An unfortunate and preventable situation may arise where some offensive statement or behaviour is expressed by a group member, and is immediately pounced upon and condemned by others (perhaps even by the worker). An indication of this happening based on inadequate exploration with the person may be when he or she repeatedly attempts to interject with "But you don't understand! What I meant was . . . ," or when the person appears to give up participation in the discussion out of frustration at not being heard and feeling defeated. A policy of "zero tolerance" of certain behaviours, such as racist remarks and violence, has become popular in various settings. Surely in a social work group, where the practice is informed by knowledge and skills and objectives that relate to personal growth and change, the intent of intervention would not be to "convict without a hearing" or to intervene in a way that may preclude the possibility of new social learning. A practice example described by Abrams (2000) illustrates the patient, caring, and persevering intervention by the worker in resolving successfully an extremely conflictual situation in a group of displaced and traumatized Bosnian and Latino boys.

Exploration of the issue can be tedious, volatile, anxiety provoking, and demanding. Socialized lessons in understanding the world may have to change for some group members. This can evoke anger, guilt, defensiveness, and offensiveness, as one another's cherished family and cultural beliefs are subjected to examination and assessment in the group.

Safety, therefore, in this learning environment is essential and, to the extent possible, is the responsibility of the worker to ensure. Instead of silencing with a "no tolerance" intervention, communication channels need to be kept open for people to explain themselves and have an opportunity to question and rethink their learned views. Shutting people down for expressing an oppressive attitude leaves their views untouched and intact. An opportunity for self-examination and altering of views, empathy, and gaining of insight will be lost. As said a half century ago by Wilson and Ryland (1949/1981), "Members of a group can be understood only against their own frames of reference for values and consequent norms of behavior" (p. 37), and "It is within the group setting that values and norms receive the greatest impetus to change" (p. 40). Zero tolerance means maintenance of the status quo, except that one member is now in a position of social exclusion. Nothing will be learned to change the views or dynamics for the future, and the group and its members will have suffered a wound from which they may not recover.

6. While acknowledging the differences, there may be significant commonalities shared by the parties. Before proceeding with discussion based on the assumption of difference, the presence of shared values, attitudes, customs, beliefs, or goals should be sought. Out of our ethnospecific and otherwise personal-reference-group-specific socialization, we typically see the world as "we/they." Without opportunities to learn about similarities across reference groups and personal networks, people may hold divisive misassumptions about the uniqueness of their views. A positive result of conflict resolution may be that some of those misassumptions of difference are dispelled, that people gain an awareness of commonalities that unite rather than divide them. They also can gain greater knowledge of another culture or belief system, which may result in an enhanced sense of oneness with others in a broader social environment, and also give oneself a clearer understanding of one's own beliefs through self-examination and scrutiny by others.

We all are members of the human family, with commonalities and uniquely differentiating characteristics across people and our various groupings. The differences need to be acknowledged and respected as valid; they give society its "richness of diversity." The commonalities also, however, need to be brought to light in order for people to recognize the common elements of their respective history, beliefs, customs, and

struggles. New awareness of previously unknown similarities can elimi-
nate an internecine competition for status and resources, and initiate
among the members a spirit of collective action against oppressive and
problematic conditions for the good of all. Group membership should
mean inclusion, not assimilation, of differences.

7. Creating an awareness of "centrism" may be an important part
of the group worker's intervention. Centrism is an exclusive focus on
one's own reality, with assessment of others' differences ranked
in relation to one's own reference groups. In the course of lifelong
socialization within particular reference groups, people learn the
characteristics of their own personal identity groups within the context of the groups' life experiences, worldview, larger culture, beliefs,
values, attitudes, assumptions, and social location. A middle-age,
Canadian-born, heterosexual woman of Irish Catholic heritage has
received different social learning and will have a different self-
concept, set of understandings of the world, and sense of belonging in
personal reference groups than a young gay man who has immigrated
recently to North America from Vietnam.

It may be argued that centrism, in that one has a solid sense of who
one is, is appropriate and necessary. The dangerous aspect of centrism, however, may come in setting one's own social identity groups'
characteristics as the benchmark by which others are evaluated. An
"I/you–we/them" dynamic is put into operation, loaded potentially
with discrimination against those deemed "other." The implication in
messages can be that these are not just the ways of "our country" or
"our religion," but that our ways are *the* way. We humans seem to be
programmed to rank differences, which from a centric vantage point
can mean that "our" place in the social arena is at the top, and all "others" fall into their places of worth and status or legitimacy somewhere
below. Inclusion of "other" ways as "also valid" can be an effective
step in resolving the cognitive and affective aspects of experiencing
conflict as an expression of difference. Centrism is a mind-set built on
socially created divisions of difference that get ranked: all "others"
against the benchmark. Get rid of the benchmark mentality. See and appreciate difference in people's socially learned beliefs and attitudes and
history, but without the ranking. Difference is difference, a parallel social
phenomenon, not a vertical power differential.

8. Integral in reshaping one's worldview to include fair consideration of differences in others is the thoughtful practising of respect.

Effective as modelling, the group worker's intervention must be characterized by respect. When we say we conduct our lives and professional careers according to values that honour and affirm the intrinsic worth, human rights, and dignity of all people, it means that we operate with a worldview and practice approach of inclusivity, rather than separation and exclusion of some people. Otherwise, what we do may negate what we say we value about people.

9. Language is a powerful conveyor of subtle and blatant messages of values and meaning. Our choices of words and attention given in a group to words used by group members are significant indicators of underlying attitudes and beliefs. Language literally and ideologically says it all. What is the message of regard expressed when people are called by an adjective, like "the poor," "the disabled," instead of people who are poor or who have a disability, or when an alternative practice modality to group work is referred to as "one *on* one"? Unfortunately, it may not be uncommon to hear in a group, "Well, he's a [fill-in-the-blank], you know what they're like," as if "they" all are clones. The wholeness and uniqueness of individuals is neither acknowledged nor respected. The group worker can monitor and raise for analysis messages of disrespect, and/or misassumption or misunderstanding of difference, especially noting those that are unintended, unconscious, or implicit.

10. Acknowledging difference means gain not loss. If the members of a social work group are regarded as a pool of resources available to contribute to the tasks of the group for the benefit of all, differences among the members represent a broader base of knowledge and experience to apply to the work. The group is better able to undertake its purposes. Garland, Jones, and Kolodny (1978) refer to the fourth stage of group development, differentiation, in which "we see emerging a new acceptance of individual differences and . . . free expression in this regard" (p. 53). At this stage, "[a] range of difference among the members is valued as important for enriching the experience. As they assume more responsibility for sharing their perceptions and conflicts, these feelings are more readily accepted as essential for the problem-solving process" (Glassman and Kates, 1990, p. 95). Differences are an asset, not a liability, in achieving group purposes.

EXAMPLES AND DISCUSSION OF GROUP CONFLICT ARISING FROM DIFFERENCE

The following are four examples of conflict arising in a group, sparked by a perception of difference and a reaction of antagonism and opposition. Discussion with reference to the practice principles for desirable conflict accompanies each one.

Vignette 1. Mixed Teen Group in a Child Protection Agency: Difference of Perspective and Experience That Gets Ranked

Laura makes the statement that people who have "ok families" complain about little things, but don't know what bad families really are like. The worker attempts to get her to talk about her family by asking about her father. Nazra says she'd rather be hit than subjected to the embarrassment her stepfather causes her by coming to her school drunk, and talking to her friends. Both Kenny and Laura emphatically say that's not worse than being hit. Laura refers to the difficulty explaining bruises on her arms and legs. Kenny says he "fell off his bike" a lot. Laura adds that she got pushed down the stairs, but says her parents were very careful—they'd hit her on her back, or on her legs in the winter when they were covered with tights, places where people couldn't see. Nazra initially attempts to stay in the discussion, then appears exasperated, and withdraws into silence.

The young people here are in conflict over their differing perceptions of what describes a bad family. Both differences and commonalities are expressed as Laura and Kenny establish an alliance with each other in their shared criterion of physical abuse, and Nazra is put aside on the basis of her different view. All these disclosures flow freely, though expressed with pain, from the group members, each leading into the next. The result of the difference is that Nazra, who initially had triggered Laura's statement, is left feeling put down, and her experiences invalidated. In the social interaction, Nazra is excluded from the base of common ground shared by Laura and Kenny. This especially is a loss for Nazra, as she previously had been allied with Kenny on many occasions.

Possible worker intervention may have served to help name and explore the similarities across the circumstances of all the group members present towards a composite list of characteristics of bad families assembled from the experience of all of them. What happens here is an assessing and ranking dynamic that excludes one member at a time when she has risked herself by disclosing difficult personal information. Monitoring the content and interaction, the worker might have commented to the group as a whole, "It sounds like there's more than one way a family can be bad. Kenny and Laura and Nazra have told us about their firsthand knowledge of how a bad family can be. Kenny and Laura know about hitting and physical violence, and Nazra knows about being embarrassed by her stepfather when he's drunk and goes to her school. In what other ways can a family be bad?" (The worker is scanning the group and attempting to make eye contact with each member as these invitational words are spoken.) In whatever responses follow from the teens, the worker would be listening for references to commonalities and reframing personal or specific examples from members into conceptualized characteristics to which all the members can relate. Examples of commonly agreed on descriptors may be "families that make a kid feel ashamed (or hurt, or unloved, or unwanted, or afraid)," "families that do things that make it hard for kids to do their schoolwork (or have friends)," or "families that make kids feel that there's something wrong with them (or that they have caused the family's problems)." When a range of examples is given, the worker's task is to de-emphasize (but not deny) the individual differences, and attempt to help the members ally with one another in their similar feelings about being kids in bad families and what that means for them.

Vignette 2. Mixed Teen Group in a Child Protection Agency: Difference of Attitude

Dwight says, "One day I grabbed my dad's stereo cause he got mad at me, and I started throwing it everywhere. He grabbed a knife and whipped it at me. The handle hit me in the back of the neck." Kenny says, "You don't beat up on people . . . say you had a kid, . . . well, if I had a kid, I wouldn't hit my kid, right?" Dwight retorts in a surly and belligerent tone, "I'm not that dumb, I'm not dumb." Kenny persists, "But if you're raised up in an abusive household, it might happen, right? But you try and make it better than it was for you?" Dwight mumbles, looking physically uneasy, and sidesteps the issue by making a comment about sitting on a cockroach.

A difference in attitude about the continuation of family violence into the next generation is expressed here between Kenny and Dwight, with Kenny's concern and projection into the future met with a tone of aggression from Dwight. Both boys have known physical and emotional abuse in their families. Dwight is caught in the culture of family violence, and participates in it. Kenny has moved to a view that family violence is wrong and will not be part of his future. Dwight initially reacts with words conveyed with a threat of aggression towards Kenny, then backs down and averts the issue.

Here is an opportunity for the group worker to confront the difference expressed by the boys and to assist them and the other members in exploring the effects of family violence on them, and in advancing their thinking towards their future possibilities with families of their own. As it was, Dwight responds to Kenny's earnest vision initially with a retort veiled in aggression and defensiveness. Although Kenny proceeds with his point, Dwight cannot participate with him. The worker, perhaps, could have intervened to empathize with Dwight, diffuse his anger towards Kenny, and access his pain: "You know, I think Kenny's got a point here that you all may have some thoughts about. At the same time, though, if kids grow up with violence as a regular part of their family, it could be kind of hard to think of doing it differently yourself some day. What do you all think about that?" (The worker scans the whole group, with particular and warm regard towards Dwight.)

The hoped-for ensuing discussion could be useful in drawing in other members, validating and reinforcing Kenny's positive and sensible attitudes, and instilling hope in Dwight and the others that despite the overwhelming discouragement experienced in common in their current situations, their futures may be better through their own doing. *Now* doesn't have to be *always*. The opportunity for all members to relate to these concerns may be beneficial for each one individually with regard to the content, and as well to the evolution of a sense of groupness, in highlighting the shared aspects of a daunting reality with present and future implications.

Vignette 3. Social Work Student Group: Difference of Ethnicity

In a foundations course in a BSW program, a small group of students has the task of researching, preparing, and delivering to the class a presentation on employment issues. Early in their discussion, types of work arise as a topic, including that done outside and within the home. These bright students, all women and of mixed ages, then move to the implications of gender and cultural prescriptions and customs. The issue arises of a woman's availability to work outside the home when older family members require care. One of the students, Hindu from India, states, "Well, in *my* culture, we care about our old people and take care of them at home." Another retorts, "It's not just your culture. I'm from Portugal, and *we* would never put our parents or grandparents in an old age home." The first one argues back about *her* culture, as if disbelieving the second student, and a third student then pipes up with the revelation, "I've got news for you two. *My* family came from Ireland, and we think the same as you about taking care of our aging relatives." Some prickly verbal exchange takes place, including some disparaging comments about "Canadians" not feeling the same care or responsibility towards their families as people of other cultures. Suddenly, a fourth woman bursts into the discussion, "I don't know how you all got your ideas about Canadians, but I'm Canadian, and my parents have lived with me and my husband and our children for almost twenty years!" Her interjection has the effect of stopping the action for a moment. Then comes the huge, simultaneous realization for all of them that the custom of caring for the elderly generation in one's family does not belong exclusively to any particular culture. The women appear to revel in this newly and unexpectedly discovered sameness and unity.

With all their perceived differences, expressed with pride and vehemence, these four women discover a significant thread of commonality, which unites them across lines of values, gender, and family life. Not only is the conflict resolved in the present moment, but new social learning occurs for each person. Cultural misassumptions are corrected and negative cultural attitudes are dispelled. The sense of groupness among the women is strengthened considerably at this time, which no doubt enhances the process and product of their assignment, and, in addition, affects positively their understanding and appreciation of others' cultural ways, and their new feeling of similarity to and connection with other cultures. The specific unifying theme discovered by these women is not their cultural differences in caring for older relatives, but the gender and family commonalities across their cultures.

Thompson (1997) describes the need for an integrated approach to understanding multiple realities by citing two authors who advocate its application. Mama (1991, in Thompson, 1997, p. 11) writes: "Race, class, and gender and so on are separated out for analytical purposes, but they are not entirely separate processes; they occur simultaneously and affect people in combination. They are related dimensions of our complex existence rather than discrete entities." Williams (1991, in Thompson, 1997, p. 12) expands the identifying characteristics for analysis of multiple realities and oppressions by including age, disability, and sexuality and urges that the power and inequality patterns of social arrangements be the focus rather than individual differences, which can lead to a "hierarchy of oppressions," and needless and artificial division among people. Although Thompson's stance addresses anti-oppression social work practice in a more politicized sense, there is relevance for its application here in this vignette in his agreement with Mama and Williams in advocating an integrated approach to provide an understanding of "both the common themes across areas [of multiple and multifaceted human experiences] and the key differences between them" (Thompson, 1997, p. 12).

Vignette 4. A Men's "Anger Management" Group: Difference of Socially Learned Behaviour

There are eight men in this group. All are required to attend by the authority of the correctional system due to assault convictions against their female partners. Tension has been brewing over the past couple of sessions as a number of the men are beginning to understand the notion of the discrepant power relations between genders that characterizes many cultures, and the resulting discrimination against women that occurs in the various institutions of society, including the marital relationship. Tom and Andy frequently have found themselves agreeing on their views about male superiority, the "natural" way of life. They've been known to say things like, "There are certain things about life that just are, and always have been! Like it or lump it!" In this session, Dan, a member who initially was allied with Tom and Andy, states that he now can sort of imagine how the relationship dynamics between him and his partner, Sally, must have been for her. He compares how he remembers feeling when, as a boy, he was outpowered by his father and frustrated beyond words with an unspeakable combination of fear, desperation, self-loathing, and rage. As Dan relates this to the group, his face and voice soften into tears. Andy reacts by standing, and lunging toward Dan with his finger pointing at him, saying, "You can be a limp dick if you want, but you're not going to make me one. I'm a man, and I'm proud of it. That's how I was raised and it's the way it's supposed to be. [And as he turns to the worker] Do you hear me? Why are you and these "foreigners" trying to say it's wrong? I was born here, and I know what's right. The man's the man, and the woman's the woman. It's even in the Bible." With that, a usually quiet member, Fred, stands up to Andy and says, "Look, we're trying hard to fix things in our lives. You don't seem to fit. I think you should leave!" Several of the men join in the conflict, standing and shouting back and forth, Andy versus all the others.

The group worker in this setting may feel like volunteering to be the one to leave. The prospect of reshaping this situation into a positive social learning experience may seem unlikely, but that objective may be possible and would be desirable. The competing forces of sexist and egalitarian gender relations could hardly be presented more explicitly and accessible for intervention than what occurs in the live group process generated among these men.

Respect will be a central ingredient in the worker's intervention. The differing views expressed in the here and now of the group must be framed within a family and cultural tradition of beliefs and norms, which for its members are "the right way" to live. The dynamics in this group are particularly challenging in that there is an uneven progression of change in the personal views among the men. Those who recently have gained insights about themselves and have learned new lessons about gender and behaviour may be both zealous and fragile in their new understandings. Their views of themselves and the organization and operations of society have transformed, and there is a tendency to blame or criticize a member who is still at the place from which they have moved. Blaming, however, will negate intended messages of respect. In order to minimize the tendency to blame Andy for his views (which all held until very recently), the worker may invite a sharing of views, generalized, for example, as "conventional male socialization": the lessons learned across many cultures about male superiority and dominance.

Although it may seem that Andy has said enough to make his views quite clear, further exploration is indicated. Andy needs an opportunity to describe how his understandings and attitudes originated, and how they have been meaningful in his life. In addition, the group needs an opportunity for all members to connect with Andy, to see themselves in him, and to gain further insight into the effects of sexist views on their relationships, self-image, and concept of "maleness," and perhaps on the resulting nature of wider society as well.

As the group worker will empathize with all present around the socialization lessons that the men have learned involuntarily, and the costs incurred in relationships for their male privilege, he or she also will assist the members to recognize their commonalities, a major one possibly being the hope of enjoying life better with the people they love. Helping the men see multiple bases for empathizing with one another may be the operative dynamic in their becoming a system of mutual care, support, and aid.

The eruption of conflict as an expression of difference in a social work group is a gift to the worker and members. It is a slice of real life, which, although creating some raw and challenging moments, provides an opportunity to take stock of one's views, and through reassessing them under the lens of peers, to choose to broaden or alter one's perspective. A group in social work practice still can be a means of continuing socialization lessons in order to enhance individuals' personal life experience, and to prepare them with attitudes and competencies to contribute in their personal networks. Every personal change that results in someone becoming fairer and more respectful, thoughtful, understanding, and egalitarian in his or her regard for other people changes the nature of the greater society. This is a way in which those important behavioural and ideological advances can happen, and social group work can be a useful means of their realization.

REFERENCES

Abrams, B. (2000). Finding common ground in a conflict resolution group for boys. *Social Work with Groups, 23*(1), 55-69.

Bernstein, S. (1978). Conflict and group work. In S. Bernstein (Ed.), *Explorations in group work: Essays in theory and practice* (pp. 72-106). Bloomfield, CT: The Practitioner's Press.

Coyle, G. L. (1959/1980). Some basic assumptions about social group work. In A. S. Alissi (Ed.), *Perspectives on social group work practice: A book of readings* (pp. 36-51). New York: The Free Press.

Garland, J. A., Jones, H. E., and Kolodny, R. L. (1978). A model for stages of development in social work groups. In S. Bernstein (Ed.), *Explorations in group work: Essays in theory and practice* (pp. 17-71). Bloomfield, CT: The Practitioner's Press.

Glassman, U. and Kates, L. (1990). *Group work: A humanistic approach*. Newbury Park, CA: Sage Publications, Inc.

Goroff, N. N. (1972). Unique properties of groups: Resources to help people. *Child Welfare, 51*(8), 495-504.

Hirayama, H. and Hirayama, K. (1986). Empowerment through group participation: Process and goal. In M. Parnes (Ed.), *Innovations in social group work: Feedback from practice to theory* (pp. 119-131). Binghamton, NY: The Haworth Press.

Kaiser, C. A. (1958/1980). The social group work process. In A. S. Alissi (Ed.), *Perspectives on social group work practice: A book of readings* (pp. 52-63). New York: The Free Press.

Klein, A. F. (1970). *Social work through group process*. New York: School of Social Welfare, State University of New York at Albany.

Kurland, R. and Salmon, R. (1998). *Teaching a methods course in social work with groups*. Alexandria, VA: Council on Social Work Education, Inc.

Mondros, J. B., Woodrow, R., and Weinstein, L. (1992). The use of groups to manage conflict. *Social Work with Groups, 15*(4), 43-57.

Simmel, G. (1955). *Conflict and the web of group-affiliations.* New York: The Free Press.

Somers, M. L. (1962). Helping through social group work: An introductory statement. In *Potentials for service through group work in public welfare* (pp. 1-4). Chicago: American Public Welfare Association.

Steinberg, D. M. (1997). *The mutual-aid approach to working in groups: Helping people help each other.* Northvale, NJ: Jason Aronson, Inc.

Thompson, N. (1997). *Anti-discriminatory practice.* London: The Macmillan Press Ltd.

Wilson, G. and Ryland, G. (1949/1981). *Social group work practice: The creative use of the social process.* Hebron, CT: The Practitioner's Press.

Chapter 6

Putting Social Justice on the Agenda: Addressing Habitual and Social Barriers

Paule McNicoll

The mind sees only what it is looking for and is only looking for what it has in mind.

Anonymous

INTRODUCTION

Paradigms, theories, models, and frameworks are basic tools of perception, assessment, and evaluation. Currently, most social work agencies are working from an extended medical model sometimes called the biopsychomedical model. It is a residual model: involvement is exclusively reserved to problematic situations. And while social work agencies often profess to adhere to ecological systems theory, the practice they support still tends to address problems at the individual and nuclear-family level and to pay lip service to analyses and interventions at the collective, community, and societal levels. In this chapter, I will pose that the current vision of social work limits the practice of social work in general, and more specifically the practice of social group work. I will propose some preliminary ideas towards the creation of a new framework that would aim at the reorganization of society for the benefit of all citizens through the enhancement of social cohesion and participation, and the recognition and mobilization of people's strengths and resources. This new formulation of social work practice would have the potential to bring back the social in social work and permit group workers to reclaim the rightful place they have lost over the years through the myopic practice of individualizing social problems and separating problems from elements of solution. Before I do this, however, I will invite the readers to share the path I followed to the realization that something was amiss in the organization of social work practice.

My quest started a year ago in Toronto when I was invited to do an inventory of innovative social work with groups to address issues of social justice. I found more socially progressive group work activity than I expected, but, to my surprise, only in a minority of cases were these groups facilitated by social workers. Even more surprising was the fact that, while social work students were very active in facilitating such groups, they tended to stop doing work aimed at social change once they graduated. A few years after the completion of their degrees, most of our social development graduates had found employment in professional agencies, particularly in child protection and hospitals, and their practice focused on counseling and practical intervention at the individual and familial levels. If we make an exception for the work of several academics (e.g., Breton, 1989; Cohen and Mullender, 1999; Gutiérrez, Parsons, and Cox, 1998; Lee et al., 1997; Lordan, 2000; Salazar, 1991), the few social work graduates who continued with progressive social work with groups were working in nongovernmental agencies that specialize in social development, sometimes locally, sometimes in developing countries. Most, if not all of them, worked for a pittance.

I am not saying that it is not possible to do progressive work in institutional settings, but it is much more difficult, requires advanced, sometimes almost subversive, skills, and therefore is relatively rarely done. For me, the evidence was clear: by and large, professional social work institutions are not promoting and sponsoring groups that work for social justice. In fact, these institutions may even impede progressive and emancipative work. Reflecting on this unexpected finding, I came to discover that there were structural barriers to the creation of groups that aim towards social justice. All was not bleak, however. On the positive side, there were also some recent developments that presented opportunities for group workers.

BARRIERS

In my survey, I identified three barriers to social group work practice: a residual model of social work service delivery, social workers' habit of conceptualizing social work, and the isolation of people who do social justice work. The first one is by far the most important barrier. The other two are the consequences of the first, although they are also barriers in their own right.

Residual Social Service Model

Social workers are operating in a service model that is overwhelmingly residual as opposed to preventive and inclusive. In other words, our profession has adopted a medical model of practice in which people have to be labeled as "having a problem" to access service. By and large, social workers work with people who have problems—no identified problem, no access to the services of a social worker. There are two main career paths towards becoming a social work client: either one is identified as having a problem by some kind of authority, mostly through the court system, and is mandated to take a minimum dose of social services treatment, or one self-identifies as needing help. In both cases, the individual is judged to be deficient in dealing with a certain type of situation. The labeling exercise having happened at the micro level, it follows that the work would also be done at that level. Thus, the focus of intervention is the individual (or the family), and not the situation and/or environment.

The residual model is similar to the medical model in medicine. Its residual organization is based on the premise that it is less expensive to address problems than to promote wellness. This is a debatable and debated argument. Proponents of a more holistic model make the point that it would be less expensive, in the long run, to prevent problems rather than address them when they have fully developed. However, the purse holders are the politicians who are elected for four years and are made accountable for the state of their financial administration within that period. The decision makers realize that, in the short run, it would be more costly to pay for both the resolution of current problems and the prevention of future ones. The worse off the economy, the less likely a change towards a holistic model of social services is to be. The choice of a residual model is also supported by the philosophy that citizens should not depend on the state for their well-being, and that only in the last resort should the state provide services that could interfere with people's private lives.

Unfortunately, there are implications for our adoption of this model. First and most obvious is the implicit mandate that individuals need to adapt to their environment and not the other way around. Many social workers resist this focus on changing the person and include advocacy and empowerment in their work. But in a system organized around the notion of deficiency, with most clients already having bought that notion and expecting individualized help, it becomes problematic at many levels to turn the problem around and work for some form of social change. Second, with a focus on problems rather than on the whole-system person/environment, it is also easy to forget that people are more than just their problems, but that they are also dynamic and resourceful. It is less likely in problem-focused groups that the facilitators will heed Margot Breton's admonition to listen to lessons from the past in regard to working holistically with clients. Breton (1990) wrote, "A group can be structured so that only the hurt, broken, troubled part of the person is invited, but it can also be structured so that the whole person in each member is invited" (p. 27).

Obviously, she meant that the latter situation is the preferred one. And that one revictimizes the person when one recognizes only the problem, and not the full human being. (To be fair, it is still possible to invite the full person in the present system, but it is more difficult because it involves intentionally changing the tacit contract existing between institution and client.) Third, the energy level of people who face difficulties tends to be lower than when they are in full form. Thus, a group of people selected on the basis of having coping problems will find fewer resources available at any one point than a regular group of citizens. Finally, besides being reductive in scope, the residual model is also reductive in terms of time. Social work services are perceived as expensive (and they are when working one-on-one), and agencies often limit the period of contact between client and social worker. One has barely addressed the current crisis before it is time to close the case. There is little to no time for consciousness raising, even though Judith Lee and other proponents of empowerment practice consider it "unethical to 'treat' victims clinically and interpersonally without attempting to help them raise consciousness, throw their oppressors off their backs and become victors" (Lee, 1997, p. 18).

The residual model of service is an important structural barrier that brings with it two consequences that are also barriers in their own right: our own habits of conceptualizing social work and the isolation of people who do social justice work.

Social Workers' Habit of Conceptualizing Social Work

Working within a reductive system day in and day out, we unconsciously adopt its underlying conceptualization of social work and accompanying habits of work. When I was invited to work with a community of Vietnamese older people in 1993, I promptly designed a close-ended traditional support group for eight to twelve people who were supposed to meet with two facilitators for eight weeks. In no uncertain terms, these people made me realize that they wanted none of this program. They wanted, and got, a permanent large group where they could get information, education, language training, recreation, and the freedom to organize for the betterment of their and other people's lives (McNicoll and Christensen, 1995). They wanted the kind of nurturing milieu provided by settlement houses. These Vietnamese people saw themselves as a collectivity of citizens, and they rightly rejected the attempt I made to "individualize" their process of adaptation in their new country.

An observation I want to share as an aside is that it appears that our mode of structuring social services seems to be restricted to so-called developed countries. When social workers work in the developing world, there is no questioning the preponderance of the social development model. Why is social work practice in these two worlds so different? I don't have an answer to that, other than to point out two avenues for further thought: one, the Western tendency to perceive people as individuals independent from their social milieu, and, two, the tendency to perceive people living very different lives in more abstract and generic terms. The latter tendency would then explain why we devise generic programs for these people rather than more individually tailored services, the way we do for people living in North America. Of course, it is possible that the only necessary explanation is that the individualized therapeutic mode of operating would be rejected in many countries on the grounds that they are demeaning and pointless.

The Isolation of People Who Do Social Justice Work

Two years ago, a group of social work students doing social development work in five different contexts decided to start a support group for themselves. Meeting with them weekly, I heard them talk about how useful it was for them to work together because they felt so isolated and have nobody to consult with when the group process and/or the external political process becomes difficult. I invited them to attend the group workers' network we are starting in Vancouver. Their reaction was interesting: they did not perceive themselves as group workers, although they all worked with small groups of citizens. They had seen the ads for the network, but they thought they were addressed to "therapists." And when they attended the first meetings, they were indeed a bit confused by the therapeutic language of the majority of other group workers. Fortunately, social workers working in institutions decided to extend the welcoming mat and alternate the focus of our meetings: one meeting on work based originally on social change, the next meeting on work that starts from the remedial approach. Still, I was impressed by the fact that neither group easily perceived that they had much in common. And to be frank, the coming together of these two groups is still shaky. Each group is eager to obtain skills directly relevant to its own work and shows slight impatience when the focus is on the other group. The situation may even be worse where there exists a division of the profession between social workers and community organizers, with each group having its independent professional organization.

OPPORTUNITIES

The past few years have provided us with a few opportunities for developing groups for social justice. I am talking about a quickening of theoretical models relevant to social justice groups, the growing legitimacy of participatory action research, the activity of the Theatre of the Oppressed in many urban centers, and the emergence of the health promotion model. I'll address the first three briefly and will then focus on the last one, which I consider the most likely to make a lasting difference.

A Quickening of Theoretical Models Relevant to Social Justice Groups

Of course the theoretical basis for social justice work is not new. We owe thanks to Paolo Freire, Elizabeth Lewis, Ruby Pernell, and many others. But there seems to be a quickening of recent theoretical activity for empowerment, social justice, and emancipation. I don't want to go into details, but I want to mention the work of the past decade (well, twelve years in fact): starting with Margot Breton's reconnecting group work practice with our traditions from the settlement, recreation, and progressive education movements (Breton, 1989), continuing with the development of self-directed groups by Audrey Mullender and David Ward (1991), the multifocal vision of Judith Lee (1994, 2000), and the concept of empowerment practice by Lorraine Gutiérrez, Ruth Parsons, and Enid Opal Cox (1998). Finally, I applaud the challenge to the well-established group work classification that limits the scope of group work activity by Marcia Cohen and Audrey Mullender (1999) and a new configuration of the connections among different modalities of social work with groups that encourage full development of the group potential by Margot Breton, Enid Opal Cox, and Susan Taylor (2000). The collective works of these theorists have liberated us from the confines of a too-limited vision of what can be achieved by small groups.

The Growing Legitimacy of Participatory Action Research

A second opportunity is the new legitimacy of participatory action research (PAR), which is based on Paolo Freire's work. PAR is the processing of a group of people's struggle for a better life. It generally starts with a mundane problem in daily living and a collective reflection about the sources and implications of the problem. A decision for action and the action itself follow, and a new round of reflection is initiated about the new knowledge acquired and the new configuration of daily life. PAR is a cycle of social consciousness, social action, and community building that leads to collective empowerment, personal growth, and greater social justice. Arturo Ornelas, a PAR facilitator in Mexico, states it this way:

> Participatory action research is about movement for personal and social transformation. It permits us, little by little, to discover the reality of our lives. When we as a group investigate our situation and make decisions to take power and create justice, we transform our reality. In so doing, we also are transformed— losing fear and gaining self-esteem. We build knowledge: the wisdom of the people. (In Laszlo and Norris, 1993, p. 16)

PAR is now taught in many schools of social work. It is group work and requires advanced group work skills to be done properly. By allying with our colleagues who are PAR researchers, we can help form social workers who integrate successfully research and group work skills to be used for social justice purposes.

The Activity of the Theatre of the Oppressed in Many Urban Centers

A third opportunity is the activity of the Theatre of the Oppressed, also an influence of Paolo Freire. Such theatre groups exist in many urban centers. It is called Theatre for Liberation in Seattle and Theatre for Living in Vancouver. It also is very active in Toronto.

In one form or an another, these groups organize public events that address one common problem in people's lives, why this problem exists, and how to address this problem. These performances are very powerful because they touch more than just the intellect. The new knowledge participants gain is inscribed in the body and involves the imagination. There is a live connection between those who play out roles and the members of the audience. I am personally very inspired by this work and find in it many ideas I would like to integrate in my work. I also think that there is good potential for an alliance and common work on specific issues. Theatres of the Oppressed are very active in current urban and rural struggles of interest to social workers.

The Emergence of the Health Promotion Model

A last and most critical opportunity in certain countries is the emergence of the health promotion model. In Canada and some other countries around the world (United Kingdom, Australia, Scandinavian countries), the medical model is under challenge where it hurts the most—in the health care system.

Health promotion is a universal model. Its aim is "health for all," not "curing the sick," as it would be in a residual model. Health promotion emphasizes community over individuals, focuses equally on the strengths and on the problems, and encourages community participation and mutual aid.

Health promotion is the official basis for health policy in Canada since 1986. It is also the official health policy of the World Health Organization. Of course, as we all know in Canada, the policy and the current reality have very little in common. But I perceive an opportunity there. Look at the mission statements of hospitals and community health centers—they are based on health promotion. We can use these statements to back up arguments to do different types of groups and work in more progressive ways. Some British authors (Drysdale and Purcell, 1999; Reverand and Levy, 2000) have also noted the place made for group work by the health promotion model.

A Framework for Social Work

Because, as social workers, we have adapted to working in a residual model, we seem to have forgotten to develop an alternative vision. Why not build for ourselves a model that would be similar to the framework for health promotion, a model that would aim at creating social justice and well-being for all? Here is a draft of what this could look like. Of course, there would need to be more work done on such a model, and I wouldn't dream of doing this alone. Also, unfortunately, a social justice and well-being promotion model would be unlikely to be adopted in the current economic times. Still, it wouldn't hurt to be ready when the right political and economic climates come forth.

The aim would be to attain social justice and well-being *for all*. This model would establish that social workers work for the whole society, and not only, and in passing, with people who have difficulty coping. Even if administrators and others who hire social workers are not adopting our all-encompassing view, we could still maintain, develop, and promote our vision if we had a clear and simple model to counteract the message they give us by defining so narrowly the social work job market. The model also provides us with a much wider mandate.

The *challenges* we would address are *reducing inequities,* not only a source of poor physical health, but a sure source of social malaise; *building strengths,* which would support a rationale for program-based and group-based interventions (e.g., camping, sports, education, festivals); and *enhancing coping,* which is the part that is already legitimated at present. The three challenges are complementary and can lead only to a socially healthy society when addressed at the same time and with equal vigor. For instance, enhancing coping in an unfair context is not only counterproductive but also ethically problematic.

The second level, *interventions,* identifies both the types of social work interventions that the model privileges and what can be done to move from the current residual model to the new one. If we plan to improve other people's situation, would it not be important to start by addressing the structural issues that put our profession in a vise? I will use the model to illustrate how it can contribute to an implementation of the framework for social work. The same interventions and strategies would become the proposed tenets of social work practice. *Advocacy* would mean to counter the residual model of social work service delivery and address the limited employment situation of social work graduates. This would require direct action. We would have to convince social work employers to create jobs that have both of the following characteristics: a holistic mandate and adequate remuneration. We would have to advocate for positions that use the social work role to its full extent. For this we will need to have strong arguments. A good beginning is a clear model supported by research findings. Social workers would also have to foster their own *empowerment.* Even if convincing employers takes time, the model would help social workers to avoid old habits bred through limited practice. It is often possible to push the limits of workplace constraints with a little bit of initiative. In fact, creating groups, in my experience, is probably the most efficient way to do so. But one has to have a sense of the possibilities. The model would expand the domain of the possible and fire the imagination. Finally, *fostering social support* means supporting the basic idea of society wherein individuals and groups contribute to one another's well-being in hard times as well as in good times.

On a day-to day basis, and as a place to start the work, we need to employ the following *strategies:* organizing for change, encouraging critical analysis, and fostering mutual aid. *Organizing for change* requires that we decide to implement the model and embark on the mental, cultural, practical, and political tasks ahead. One way of doing this at the same time as gaining and motivating allies is to *encourage critical analysis* at every opportunity. If we believe that social group work is the powerful and liberating tool we say it is, why don't we organize to "mine" it to its maximum by engaging in *mutual aid?* A promising avenue is to network with other group workers, making sure we are including those who are doing work complementary to ours. Then share, exchange, reflect together, learn from one another, and organize together for the full realization of the potential of social group work. The tasks presented in the model are more than merely compatible with social group work; they are its essence.

CONCLUSION

To summarize, the current organization of social work practice does not favor the creation of groups that specifically pursue social justice. Three particular barriers have been identified: the residual quality of social work service delivery, social workers' habit of conceptualizing social work at the individual and familial levels, and the isolation of the few people who are involved in social justice work. Fortunately, there are also some developments worth noticing: the development of more inclusive theoretical models, the growing popularity of participatory action research and popular theatre, and the emergence of the health promotion model. In this chapter, I proposed an adaptation of the health promotion model for social work. This model would broaden the vision of social work practice as it is currently practiced and will give social group work and, more particularly, group work that focused on social justice the due place they are now denied. If we want to reconnect with our tradition of working in settlements and towards progressive change, we have to create the vision and conditions for this work to be viable. I see it as the most urgent challenge we face in developing social groups that work towards a greater social justice.

REFERENCES

Breton, M. (1989). The need for mutual-aid groups in a drop-in for homeless women: The sistering case. *Social Work with Groups, 11,* 4: 47-61.

Breton, M. (1990). Learning from social work group traditions. *Social Work with Groups, 13,* 3: 21-34.

Breton, M., Cox, E. O., and Taylor, S. (2000). Invitational presentation at the Twenty-Second International Symposium on Social Work with Groups, Toronto, October 21.

Cohen, M. and Mullender, A. (1999). The personal in the political: Exploring the group work continuum from individual to social change goals. *Social Work with Groups, 22,* 1: 13-31.

Drysdale, J. and Purcell, R. (1999). Breaking the culture of silence: Group work and community development. *Groupwork, 11,* 3: 70-87.

Epp, J. (1986). Achieving health for all: A framework for health promotion. *Canadian Journal of Public Health, 77:* 393-430.

Gutiérrez, L., Parsons, R., and Cox, E. (1998). *Empowerment in social work practice: A sourcebook.* Pacific Grove, CA: Brooks/Cole.

Laszlo, U. and Norris, J. (1993). *From the field: Participatory action research for change.* Calgary: The PAR Trust.

Lee, J. A. B. (1994). *The empowerment approach to social work practice.* New York: Columbia University Press.

Lee, J. A. B. (1997). The empowerment group: The heart of empowerment approach and an antidote to injustice. In Parry, J. K. (Ed.), *From prevention to wellness through groupwork.* Binghamton, NY: The Haworth Press, pp. 15-32.

Lee, J. A. B. (2000). Invitational presentation at the Twenty-Second Annual International Symposium on Social Work with Groups, Toronto, October 21.

Lee, J. A. B., with My Sister's Place group members and R. A. Martin (1997). *The empowerment group in action: My Sister's Place.*

Lordan, N. (2000). Finding a voice: Empowerment of people with disabilities in Ireland. *Journal of Progressive Human Services, 11,* 1: 49-69.

McNicoll, P. and Christensen, C. P. (1995). Making changes and making sense: Social work with groups with Vietnamese older people. In Salmon, R. (Ed.), *Group work practice in a troubled society: Problems and opportunities.* Binghamton, NY: The Haworth Press, pp. 101-116.

Nosko, A. and Breton, M. (1997-1998). Applying a strength, competence and empowerment model. *Groupwork, 10,* 1: 55-69.

Reverand, E. E. and Levy, L. B. (2000). Developing the professionals: Group work for health promotion. *Groupwork, 12,* 1: 42-57.

Salazar, M. C. (1991). Young laborers in Bogota: Breaking authoritarian ramparts. In Fals-Borda, O. and Rahman, M. A. (Eds.), *Action and knowledge: Breaking the monopoly with participatory action-research.* New York: The Apex Press, pp. 54-63.

PART III:
EVOLVING GROUP WORK
EDUCATIONAL APPROACHES

Chapter 7

Using Groups to Teach the Connection Between Private Troubles and Public Issues

Toby Berman-Rossi
Timothy B. Kelly

INTRODUCTION

The matter of polarizing individual and social troubles has been a compelling and persistent part of our profession since its inception. We have often differed in our vision of the profession's mission and have been asked to choose either an individual or a social change emphasis (Reynolds, 1934; Schwartz, 1994). Our early patterns of professional method jelled into casework, group work, and community organization and planning, with each holding forth its view of our professional purpose. Should we work person by person to provide assistance with private troubles? Should the small group be the vehicle for assisting individuals with personal and environmental troubles? Or should it be the troubles themselves to which we direct our attention (Schwartz, 1985/1986). Over time, these method divisions and the association of particular foci with casework, group work, and community organization made less sense. Over time, separating what Lee (1929) described as the "cause" (social goals) and "function" (the skills of helping) aspects of the profession had less merit to practitioners and ultimately to schools of social work. Clients needed their social workers to be smart not only about their private troubles but also about the public policy and societal context that fostered the creation of the private troubles themselves. Social workers needed to hear the ways individuals, families, groups, communities, and the greater society were intimately tied together and needed the skills to work across these systems. In addition, these divisions increasingly were a distortion of what occurred in agency life. Direct practice social workers were called upon to work with individuals, families, and groups. It no longer made sense (if it ever did) to send clients to one social worker who would talk with them individually, another who would talk with them and their families, and yet another who would bring them together with others facing similar troubles, e.g., loss of a child, life-threatening illness, and the development of friendships. In addition, these discrete method designations focused workers' attention on separate aspects of clients' lives and decreased the likelihood that they would see the link between the social and psychological dimensions of the very problems they were addressing with clients.

Early in the 1970s some schools of social work tried to remedy this dichotomous thinking and professional activity, by integrating work with individuals, families, groups, and communities within a single whole (Gitterman, 2002). The importance of seeing the profession and the lives of clients whole gained momentum (Lee, 1985/1986). New generic and integrated models of practice increasingly appeared (e.g., Germain and Gitterman, 1980, 1996; Lee, 1994, 2001; Shulman, 1982, 1999). Ideas about the social worker as generalist gained strength. Students no longer would be educated for practice with individuals, or families, or groups, or communities. Rather, all would have the skills necessary to work with systems of all sizes.

Unfortunately, method integration alone was not sufficient to truly integrate individual pain and social reform. Teaching students to work across systems did not necessarily include simultaneous work with private troubles and public issues. While there was increased support for seeing the transactional nature of the relation between persons and their environments, the propensity to dichotomize work with private troubles and public issues remained strong. The old "family quarrels" (casework versus group work versus community organization) persisted.

Thesis

Schwartz (1994) suggests that "when these polarizations appear in the professional arena, they are disruptive of technical advancement" (p. 379). We agree. Not only is the development of professional skill stunted, but also service to clients becomes distorted by the separation of psychological and social aspects of their lives.

This chapter is devoted to our efforts to deal with the vexing educational challenge of educating students to develop a professional vision that integrates both private troubles and public issues. We believe that the teaching of private troubles and public issues should be integrated and infused throughout the curriculum, and not rarified. We believe this content is best set within the larger context of teaching students to find the connections between private troubles and public issues in all they do, whether they are working with individuals, families, groups, or community. As well, it is our belief that the teaching of practice with groups is the ideal content to help students learn to see the connection between private troubles and public issues and to learn the skills of addressing themselves to this connection.

Our view does not imply that group work should bear the sole burden of teaching this material, as that would further dichotomize the concept. Rather, we assert that in an integrated methods sequence group work can place a special and unique emphasis on the ways in which private troubles are expressions of public issues and all public issues are instances of private troubles. The foundation for understanding the connection can be laid when teaching practice with individuals and families, but a more accessible understanding can occur through the teaching of group work practice. Understandably beginning students are very taken by the pain of individual persons and families. The recognition of this private pain allows us to introduce the idea that for all private pain there are public issues that bear on and help create the private pain, and this will "prime the pump," serving as a foundation for helping students to clearly see the connection.

When working with individual persons or families, the *individual* problems, which are always a case in point of a larger public issue, take precedence in the minds of students. For example, when an individual client is sitting in front of a social work student discussing his or her difficulties making the welfare-to-work appointments, the *individual* pain, obstacles, or "resistance" of the client are so powerful that the student will understandably have a difficult time recognizing the public issues of poor public transportation or lack of child care. However, if a group of women begins to discuss the infrequent and unreliable bus system or lack of appropriate child care as constant obstacles to fulfilling their welfare-to-work requirements, the public nature of the women's private troubles is much more palpable for the student.

In essence, it is easier to see the public issues side of private troubles when working with groups. The collective nature of groups gives rise to shared problems of concern and it becomes easier to "add up" the individual problems and see their relation to a larger environmental picture. In addition, the power of the common ground in groups and the strength-in-numbers dynamic can be used to help students more clearly see the connection between the public and the private, as well as the importance of people acting on their own behalf. Keeping in mind the educational principle of moving from less complex to more complex, group work has a special place in curricula for helping students master the private troubles and public issues connection. As students begin to see the public issues in their work with groups, they can be pressed to more readily make parallel connections in their work with individuals.

Our approach in this chapter will be to describe the points along the curricular stream of a generic practice sequence that provide optimal teaching moments for conveying private troubles and public issues using common group work content. To this end, we present teaching tools and strategies that can be incorporated into practice curricula that make the connection explicit and will help students to integrate this important concept into their understanding of clients' troubles and help them expand their skills. Three overriding principles guide us in our work. First, we must "merge individual and social need into a single image" (Schwartz, 1994, p. 389). Second, we need to define and teach the skills of converting private troubles into public issues and public issues into private troubles, thereby showing the connections between. Finally, we must teach the practice skills for working transactionally with private troubles and public issues, in groups.

ISSUES AND CHALLENGES
FOR TEACHING AND LEARNING

We believe there are several areas to which we must address ourselves. Each of these areas offers distinctive challenges for teaching and learning that, in turn, contribute to a strategy for teaching necessary content regarding the connections between private troubles and public issues. We offer what we believe are predominant rather than exclusive patterns. These are a set of generalizations. They will not apply to all situations, all the time, but they seem to capture our experience in our community and we hope our observations have captured shared truths. We have not attempted to be exhaustive in our notations, but rather to identify those aspects we consider most salient.

These areas of examination include students, group work itself, the profession, the social agency, and the subject matter itself of using groups to teach the connection between private troubles and public issues.

Students

This involves the whole arena of who our students are, what they bring to the social work classroom and to the helping experience, and what these mean for the content. We see the following characteristics in our students:

- The propensity to individualize and to believe in individual responsibility for individual troubles, and therein an incorporation of society's dominant individualistic and deficit orientation.
- The propensity to psychologize and to offer primarily psychological explanations for behavior and social ills, reflecting society's primary explanatory mode.
- Lack of experience with social movements and distance from social cause.
- Greater professional interest in individual change than environmental change.
- Perceiving greater potency in individual rather than environmental change.
- An incorporation of the profession's dominant value system of granting higher status to working on private troubles rather than public issues.
- Preference for working with clients individually.
- An initial hesitancy toward working with groups because
  —groups are too complex;
  —too much to figure out;
  —increased uncertainty with what to do;
  —fear of not being able to hear and attend to so much simultaneously;

—the desire to limit complexity;
—favoring the individual as a means of limiting complexity and increasing a sense of accomplishment and competence;
—favoring the individual as a reflection of what is familiar;
—psychologizing and individualizing within the group decreases seeing the connection between private troubles and public issues; and
—limited appreciation of the collective, the group as a whole.

The Profession

- Dualistic thinking within the profession: work with individuals *or* with groups, *or* within the community.
- Our historic failure to see the generic elements in practice decreases our ability to see the connections between private troubles and public issues. As Lee (1985/1986) notes, this failure limits our ability to see the profession whole and people's lives whole.
- The dualism inherent within the notion of person and environment rather than person in environment.
- The separation of internal and external sources of oppression without finding the connections between the two.
- A predominant paradigm of more highly valuing individual and psychological practice.
- Systems of rewards in the profession, e.g., hierarchies of value in professional associations.
- Professional associations and licensure laws that further a separation of private troubles and public issues.
- The very invention of the concept of clinical practice, its inherent narrow definition, and our need to expend personal and environmental resources in defense of our belief in the unity between the social and the psychological.

Group Work Itself

- Debate among us concerning the major purpose of group work. We, too, discuss whether group work's purpose is individual change, social change, or some combination of the two.

- These debates are shown in our frequent characterizing of distinctive group types, e.g., therapy groups at one end and social action groups on the other.
- The separation into dichotomous group types means that groups typed as more individually focused or termed *therapy* will have greater difficulty recognizing and addressing public issues and those termed *social action* will have increased difficulty seeing and addressing private troubles, e.g., a depression group for women; a housing group focused on improving housing.
- Third-party funding for groups that focus on personal change, thus compromising work on the public issues.
- Short-term nature of groups, which focus on immediate personal change, decreases the possibility of working on private troubles and public issues.

The Agency Setting

- Within *our* community in South Florida, the prevailing worldview of clients' troubles is individualistic, psychological, and deficit-oriented.
- This prevailing worldview helps shape students' beliefs and induces individualistic, psychological, and deficit-oriented conceptions of service offerings and client need.
- The use of third-party payers of services based on the DSM-IV reaffirms this orientation.
- Applied to group work service offerings, we see the following in our community agencies:
   —group work services that are frequently short-term in nature, e.g., six to ten weeks is supposed to fix all;
   —dichotomous group types, e.g., task *or* therapy *or* social action, which by definition ruptures the connections between private troubles and public issues;
   —the dichotomizing of expressive and instrumental aspects of groups that further ruptures the connections between private troubles and public issues, e.g., a student saying, "This is a therapy group. We don't bring speakers in here";
   —groups very much focused on individual change and very focused away from the public issues that are integral to each of

these groups, e.g., anger management groups, self-esteem groups, parenting-skills groups, women's depression groups;
—a concentration of authority in the worker to direct change in fast-paced, short-term, individually oriented groups, which decrease partnership and increase the muting of clients' voices, particularly concerning the public issues that bear on the private troubles.

The Subject Matter of Using Groups to Teach the Connection Between Private Troubles and Public Issues

Finally, we want to say that our subject itself is very complex and requires considerable effort to break down the content, organize it, infuse it, and make it manageable and usable to students. Most difficult is for students to think person-in-environment so that when private troubles are identified, they naturally think environmental contributor. As well, the skills of working simultaneously on both, particularly with generalist foundation students, are difficult to teach and difficult to learn.

CONTENT

The challenges just identified help shape the infusion of content on private troubles and public issues into the group work content we ordinarily teach in the foundation and generalist curricula. Though schools place varying emphasis on group work in their curricula and there is not uniformity about the "what" or "how" of teaching group work, there is certain basic group work content that can be easily incorporated into most curricula that will help teach the connection between private troubles and public issues. These content areas are placed within the context of the phases of the helping process: history of the professional method, understanding the agency/community context, beginning phase, middle or work phase, and the ending phase.

History of Professional Method

Teaching about the history of professional method immediately introduces students to the profession's struggle with private troubles and public issues. This content provides an ideal opportunity to teach how the profession has labored with these two aspects of our lives. Though often overstated, the difference in approaches between the settlement house movement, with its social justice, environmental change, and small-group emphases, and the charity organization society movement, with its individual case-by-case emphasis, highlights the competing streams of influence within the profession. This discussion can begin to socialize students to the importance of seeing the connection.

Teaching Tool: Why You Want to Be a Social Worker

This in-class exercise begins with asking students to answer two questions in small groups: "Why did you choose social work?" and "What is your vision of social work?" The answers to the questions are then put on the board and grouped according to (1) private troubles, individual focused or deficit oriented; (2) public issues, social justice, and social change; or (3) somewhere between a person-in-environment configuration. Most students identify their desire to assist with individual change as their primary motivation. This shapes our discussion of the mission of the profession towards person-in-environment practice. In addition it identifies the devaluing of group work and allows the introduction of the power of groups.

Teaching Tool: History of Professional Method Lecture

This in-class lecture describes the history of the development of professional method by contrasting the competing streams of casework and group work. It introduces the past struggles of the profession and shows how they are still evident in today's world of practice, and it begins to socialize students to the person-in-environment perspective.

Agency Community Context

As we teach about agency and community context, we must help students see how some agencies focus primarily on the private troubles and overlook the public issues side of problems in their definition of service. We must help expand students' problem definitions. In addition, they must learn how the societal context (e.g., issues of managed care and funding) limit their attention to both sides of the equation. Likewise, helping students to understand that community services are nested in community can allow students to see the public nature of problems. Societal values and beliefs about potential members and their problems and questions about societal barriers impacting potential members should be addressed. In dealing with these issues, teachers can explicitly point out the connection and the influence on the service being offered and on the lives of the members. As well, this is an ideal place to link diversity and the differential provision of service.

Teaching Tool: Agency Fair

In this exercise students are given a brief case description of a family experiencing a significant life stressor with which most students in South Florida would be familiar. Students are then divided into groups representing the mother and child and four different types of agencies, representing a range of possible services (e.g., community centers, family counseling, mental health services, after-school programs) and orientations (e.g., individual, family, group, and deficit or strengths based). The family member group must identify what needs they have and the agencies identify what services they could provide this family. The family then goes around the room and "interviews" each agency. This exercise illustrates agency influence on problem definition, and that problem definition influences and may limit helping actions. Finally, it illustrates the problem of dichotomizing public issues and private troubles.

Beginnings

In the unit on beginnings we infuse private troubles and public issues content into the following areas: tuning in, contracting, group planning, and assessment.

Tuning In

In teaching students to tune in to the feelings and concerns members may have about a group service, teachers can guide them to imagine, not only the personal feelings and concerns, but also the ways these concerns and feelings emanate from the associated public issues, e.g., taboo societal themes can induce a sense of shame, thereby increasing reluctance to reveal feelings about taboos. Tuning in to the connection between social and psychological aspects of clients' concerns will help them "hear" the connection between the two.

Contracting

Contracting with groups involves important group work skills. It involves a definition of group purpose, worker roles, member roles, and the process for work. Including Lee's (2001) notion of empowerment as a necessary part of the contracting process provides a segue into private troubles and public issues. Contracting should, at the least, allow for the understanding of the public influence on the troubles bringing members to the group. For example, students could learn to ask, "What outside yourself contributed to having this particular problem?" During the initial contracting-with-groups lecture, students learn that they must reach for the common ground among members, hear and voice multiple themes, and reach for public influences on members' private troubles and include these connections into a working agreement.

Teaching Tool: Group Contracting Process Recording. Students are provided with a group process recording from Schwartz (1968). This process recording presents the first three meetings of a group for adolescent boys in foster care. The public policy issues concerning foster care are inherent in the boys' discussion. As the class analyzes the worker's three separate attempts to make a statement that will help the boys begin their work, we help students identify the public issues inherent to the boys' private pain. We note the reluctance of the worker to identify the public issue of foster care.

Group Planning

Group planning provides significant opportunities to teach the connection between private troubles and public issues. Two typical planning areas are especially filled with opportunity. These are group purpose and member need.

Teaching about the importance of a clear group purpose is fraught with challenges and instances for teaching about the link between private troubles and public issues. Quite often group purpose is dichotomized along instrumental *or* expressive *or* psychoeducational lines. Students must be taught that psychological and social issues are inherent in all groups and in all members' experiences, and that the potential to address both is often limited by dichotomous definitions of group purpose and type. There must be room in "therapy" groups for the inherent public issues. Likewise there must be room in "instrumental, social action, or task" groups to work on the associated private troubles. To proceed otherwise is to deny the reality of human experience.

The idea of forming a group around the identification of unmet need provides a window of opportunity to infuse private troubles and public issues content into our teaching. Too often students try to form groups without a clear recognition of a felt need among a group of people. Helping students to identify a common felt need and personal, interpersonal, and environmental stressors which generate that need will point to the connections between public and private issues.

Teaching Tool: Group Planning Exercise. Kurland and Salmon's (1998, pp. 24-27) pregroup planning exercise works beautifully in helping students develop the skills of creating a new group service. They identify planning in eight different arenas: need, purpose, composition, structure, content, pregroup contact, agency context, and social context. Using their basic exercise, we add questions about the connection between the social and psychological worlds of the clients. The purpose of their generic pregroup planning exercise is designed to increase students' skills in planning groups. Infused private troubles and public issues content is highlighted where integrated in the following outline:

1. Have the class break up into groups of four or five students and brainstorm and compile a list of everything a worker should think about, make decisions about, and do between conceiving of an idea for a group and actually holding the first meeting. After they brainstorm, ask for one item on their lists (go around the room until the answers are exhausted), and as they give their items put them into columns on the board according to these categories:
    a. *Need*—What wants drives, problems, issues, or areas of concern exist among those in the target population? *Identify both the private troubles and the associated public issues. Is there*

a visible and sufficient common ground among the members and between the private troubles and public issues?

b. *Purpose*—What are the hopes, expectations, and objectives each member has about participation? What are the ends and objectives the group will collectively pursue? *How has the group been characterized? To what extent are private troubles and public issues incorporated? Are they fused or dichotomized?*

c. *Composition*—Number and characteristics of members and workers. *Does group composition foster connections and a strong common ground or does it represent an obstacle to members seeing connections among them and between the private troubles and public issues?*

d. *Structure*—What arrangements need to be made to facilitate the work (especially time and place)? *How will time, length of group, and open- or close-ended nature affect work on private troubles and public issues?*

e. *Content*—To what will the members direct their attention? On what will they work? *To what extent are psychological and social aspects of clients lives incorporated?*

f. *Pregroup contact*—How will you recruit members and how will they be prepared? *To what extent are private troubles and pubic issues linked as part of recruitment?*

g. *Agency context*—How will agency policy, mandate, and mission impact the group? *In particular, how does the agency's context influence attention to private troubles and public issues?*

h. *Social context*—What larger social and political forces may impact the offering of a group service? *What are some of the public issues that bear on delivering the service of this group?*

2. Students are then asked to use Kurland and Salmon's pregroup planning model in small groups. Each group takes one of the following scenarios and plans a group service according to the previous items. After working on this (for about forty-five minutes) students present their plan to the class. Students must assign age, class, sexual identity, gender, and ethnicity to group members.

   a. Several members of a senior center have recently had an adult child die.

   b. Recently, several HIV-positive mothers with young children have begun to use the services of an AIDS information and treatment agency.

   c. Several participants in a community-based agency serving youth have parents with AIDS.

   d. Several seventh graders who are new to a junior high school appear to be lonely, scared, and unable to make friends.

   e. An increasing number of young adults being treated in a public mental health agency are there because of court-mandated attendance for alcohol and drug offenses.

To infuse content, (1) deductively we can ask students to be attentive to both private troubles and public issues, (2) inductively we can see how they develop their groups and then work with what they develop regarding private troubles and public issues, or (3) we can develop a combination of the two.

Assessment

Assessment and its place in social work practice has been one of the defining features of many of the professional battles in which social work educators and practitioners have engaged. Regardless of the particular "school" to which one ascribes, assessment requires the "the collection of relevant information, its systematic organization, and the analysis and synthesis of the data" (Germain and Gitterman, 1996, p. 101). When teaching students to assess the members of their groups and the group as a whole, teachers should construct questions and assignments that also include inquiry into the social and political context of the helping encounter and problems addressed. In addition, students must learn to assess the extent to which public issues bear on the private troubles of the group and its members and their ability to work on public issues.

Teaching Tool: Stages of Group Development Lecture

When presenting content on stages of group development, students are taught to assess the group's stage of development and how psychological and social issues affect that development. In addition, as the group develops, the group as a whole influences individual behavior, thus strengthening the members' abilities to work on the public issues attendant to their private troubles. Finally, students can see how the effort it takes to develop their group as a whole is a microcosm of efforts needed to foster social change in the larger society.

Middle or Work Phase

After teaching students the skills of beginnings, our second semester's curriculum moves to the work phase of helping individuals, families, and groups. Regardless of how a school organizes its curriculum, teachers should look for the specific ways to include content on private troubles and public issues that are inherent in their curricular organization. In our school we have realized that each problem domain we address in the work phase offers unique opportunities to highlight the connection between private troubles and public issues. The connection does not have to be a major topic of instruction but can easily be integrated into the lessons taught.

Point of Entry

Students must learn to see that the initial definition of work with a group serves as a point of entry. From the initial point of entry, the group can decide to move into other spheres of work. In our curriculum we teach students to help with what Germain and Gitterman (1996) define as stressors in living. These definitions serve as the conceptual basis for framing a point of entry and include interpersonal stressors, environmental obstacles, and life transitions. Groups may begin working on a life transition, for example, moving from welfare to work, but realize a public issue may be presenting an environmental obstacle to successfully navigating the life transition. Students must be taught to help the group shift between the linked areas of work.

Teaching Tool: Group for Mothers in a Halfway House. Students are taught how a worker can move from working on life transitions, the initial point of entry, to public issues. Mondros's (2000) brief description of a group for mothers in a halfway house beautifully illustrates this. Mondros describes a group worker who runs a weekly group in a halfway house for women with small children. They are former substance abusers who have been incarcerated, and most have had children placed in care. The ostensible purpose of the group is to help the women make a successful transition back to the community, and to help them learn and practice good parenting skills. Four months into the work, the mothers start complaining that they have no place to take their children and that the little park a block away is filled with used needles and trash. The worker encourages the women to invite the police captain to their group to tell him ways they think the park can be improved. The park is eventually cleaned and patrolled, and the women begin to bring their babies there to play. Moreover, they feel wonderful about what they have achieved, and their sense of potency increases.

Problem Domains

When helping students learn how to help group members with interpersonal stressors that occur within groups, a simple question about the environmental influences on the interpersonal stressor can beautifully illustrate the effect of public issues on what is occurring within their groups. A case in point involves one student who described a maladaptive pattern of communication she noticed in her group. She described a pattern of members' resistance to considering leisure skills training for boys who were in trouble in school. She kept pressing the adolescent boys to consider alternative leisure activities. The more she pushed, the more they ignored or laughed at her. When she was asked to examine what community, societal, or political forces may be contributing to this power struggle between the members and her, she realized that the boys lived in a very poor area with no recreational services at all. Sharing this realization with the boys at the next meeting promoted the group's work on the many impinging public issues in their lives.

Another problem domain in which we teach group work skills is environmental obstacles. This problem area is rich with opportunities to teach the connection between personal pain and environmental stressors. Quite often students psychologize problems that are inherently environmental. Teaching students to link personal stress with environmental stressors and then to find ways for their groups to work on the environmental obstacle goes a long way toward teaching the power of understanding the nature of private troubles and public issues.

Teaching Tool: Process Recording from Floor Group in Nursing Home. The purpose of this middle phase piece of process (fifth session) is to teach students to both hear and work with the connection between private troubles and public issues. In this example, the student worker individualizes, psychologizes, and, for the most part, fails to recognize the process of mutual aid among the men. In the process of psychologizing environmental concerns, the student misses entirely the institutionally based issue with which the men are grappling. In the classroom we have students analyze the worker's helping acts to help them recognize the psychologizing and then help them to "re-do" the worker's acts to incorporate the public issues concerns. The worker's acts are highlighted in the transcript that follows.

FLOOR GROUP IN NURSING HOME

SETTING: Home and Hospital for the Aged

GROUP MEMBERS: All males living together on a floor within a long-term care facility. Eighty percent of the members on the floor were white non-Hispanic; 10 percent were white Hispanic, and 10 percent were African American. The average age was eighty-six. All members in the following session were white non-Hispanic.

THE WORKER: A thirty-year-old, German American, first-year social work student.

THE GROUP ITSELF: The group was an open-ended floor group meeting for the thirty-one residents living on an all-male floor. The group met weekly for one-and-a-half hours. It was designed to provide an opportunity for residents to work on problems, issues, and concerns arising from institutional life and from being older persons. There was a student on the floor the year prior, but there had not been any meetings over the summer following the departure of the student. Floor groups had been in existence for only one year.

THE EXCERPT: This was the group's fifth meeting. Present were Mr. Boxer, Mr. Scher, Mr. Dodge, Mr. Livsey, Mr. Katz, Mr. Waxman, Mr. Fox, Mr. Palmer, Mr. Schwartz, and Mr. Gold. The meeting began with the residents speaking about the recent election. The group listened and talked a bit.

Mr. Dodge then introduced a problem he had at breakfast, that his food did not come up very correctly. Other members in the group said we had discussed food in this group before and that nothing gets done about it. Mr. Dodge said, "Yes, nothing can be done, nobody can get to the higher-ups. We are all helpless."

I asked him if he felt that helplessness in other things besides the food in the hospital. He replied that he did. The other men joined in and said they felt helpless about everything. Mr. Katz joined in and said, "Yes, we are very helpless; we are just here waiting for the end." Mr. Dodge said, "Yes, that's it; you just hit it right on the nose." Mr. Scher then said, "As soon as I came into the hospital, I gave up; nothing can be done."

I asked him why he had given up. He said he was old and waiting to die. Mr. Dodge then said, "That's what happens. Some of the men just don't do anything. Others want to make the most of it and others don't. That's why nobody comes to the meetings anymore."

I asked others in the group for their reactions. Most of them agreed that everybody has given up and very few of them haven't. Mr. Gold said, "If I give up, then I will die; I'll have lost everything. Have you seen it at lunchtime—when nobody talks to one another?"

I said I had eaten lunch up there the last week. He said, "You know what it's like; nobody talks to one another; there is no communication here." Mr. Dodge said, "Yes, there is just apathy everywhere," and then he pointed to Mr. Scher and said, "Look, he's given up." Mr. Schwartz, who was new to the group, said to Mr. Dodge that he eats lunch with Mr. Scher and though Mr. Scher does not say anything he enjoys eating with him.

I asked for Mr. Scher's reaction. He said he was pleased with what Mr. Schwartz said. Mr. Dodge then turned to Mr. Waxman and said, "Mr. Waxman, he is a foolish man—all he does is sing songs and clap his hands." Mr. Waxman answered, "Well, some things just don't click, you know. Anything you say to me goes in one ear and out the other."

I asked Mr. Waxman if he was angry at Mr. Dodge for saying what he said. He said "No, this man could never bother me."

Teaching Tool: Environmental Obstacle Lecture. In the unit on helping groups work on environmental obstacles, students are taught that environmental obstacles always have associated psychological consequences. Students are challenged to see the connections and be able to simultaneously work on both.

Teaching Tool: Life Transitions Lecture. Finally, in teaching students to help groups work on stressors resulting from life transitions we look for ways to teach the connection. There are many. One powerful way is to ask students to assess the strengths and limitations of the group members' environments to identify their influence on the life transition, and to develop a helping strategy to address the interplay between them.

Endings

The final unit in the integrated practice sequence concerns endings and termination. We infuse private troubles and public issues into this unit in several ways. For example, when teaching students to help the members identify future work, we discuss how work on public issues could be a part of what is identified. In addition, when short-term, individually focused groups terminate, students are asked to think about how these groups could be transformed into groups that begin working on public issues.

CONCLUSION

The false dichotomy between public issues and private troubles is deeply ingrained within our society. Numerous forces work to obscure the connections between private pain and societal influences on that pain. To counter these pervasive forces, social work educators must constantly find teaching moments to assist students to see the important connections. While the infusion should occur throughout the social work curriculum, group work offers an ideal medium for teaching the content. By outlining many of the challenges to teaching the connection between private troubles and public issues, and then offering some teaching strategies and tools, we hope to foster discussion and new study about how to better infuse the content. Who better to undertake this task than group work?

REFERENCES

Germain, C. and Gitterman, A. (1980). *The life model of social work practice.* New York: Columbia University Press.

Germain, C. and Gitterman, A. (1996). *The life model of social work practice: Advances in theory and practice* (Second edition). New York: Columbia University Press.

Kurland, R. and Salmon, R. (1998). *Teaching a methods course in social work with groups.* Alexandria, VA: CSWE.

Lee, J. A. B. (1985/1986). Seeing it whole: Social work with groups within an integrative perspective. *Social Work with Groups, 8*(4), 39-50.

Lee, J. A. B. (1994). *The empowerment approach to social work practice.* New York: Columbia University Press.

Lee, J. A. B. (2001). *The empowerment approach to social work practice: Building the beloved community* (Second edition). New York: Columbia University Press.

Lee, P. R. (1929). Social work as cause and function. In P. R. Lee (Ed.), *Social work cause and function: Selected papers of Porter R. Lee* (pp. 3-24). New York: Columbia University Press.

Mondros, J. (2001). Building resourceful communities: A group worker's guide to community work. In T. Kelly, T. Berman-Rossi, and S. Palombo (Eds.), *Group work: Strategies for strengthening resiliency* (pp. 35-50). Binghamton, NY: The Haworth Press.

Reynolds, B. C. (1934). *Between client and community: A study in responsibility in social casework.* New York: Oriole.

Schwartz, W. (1968). *Group work in public welfare.* Chicago: American Public Welfare Association.

Schwartz, W. (1985/1986). The group work tradition and social work practice. *Social Work with Groups, 8*(4), 7-27.

Schwartz, W. (1994). Private troubles and public issues: One social work job or two. In T. Berman-Rossi (Ed.), *Social work: The collected writings of William Schwartz* (pp. 377-394). Itasca, IL: F. E. Peacock Publishers (originally published in 1969).

Shulman, L. (1982). *The skills of helping individuals and groups.* Itasca, IL: F. E. Peacock Publishers.

Shulman, L. (1999). *The skills of helping individuals, families, groups, and communities.* Itasca, IL: F. E. Peacock Publishers.

Chapter 8

Restorative Education: Group-Centered Dialogue Between Students and Faculty at a Graduate School of Social Work

Stacy Husebo
Sarah Ann Schuh
Mary Beth Gustafson
Doug Beumer

Education needs to be restored by examining ideas about what, where, and how learning occurs. Lindeman (1926) viewed true education as a social process, thereby making a group-centered process an effective and exciting arena to pose questions and dialogue about issues relevant to social work education. The authors of this chapter were the main architects in creating and implementing a student-faculty dialogue that addressed responsibility in creating a liberating pedagogy. This dialogue fostered the establishment of collaborative and authentic relationships between students and faculty. The idea of restorative education, borrowed from the concept of restorative justice, seeks to restore balance and wholeness to situations by getting all voices and participants active in the education process. Education is restorative when students, faculty, and the community are the active shapers of its purpose and practice.

This chapter includes a review of the literature and a brief history of the Radical Social Work Student Group (RSWSG); describes the purpose, planning, and execution of the student-faculty forum; discusses themes that arose during the forum; addresses implications for social work practice; and offers recommendations for future dialogue.

LITERATURE REVIEW

Social work education carries the responsibility of molding future practitioners' competence and effectiveness in practice. This task is essential to create just and humane social services. Five areas of social work education are explored in this chapter: (1) ideas about education, (2) students as active shapers of their education, (3) the teacher as facilitator of the education process, (4) education as a transformational and revolutionary process, and (5) group work processes in education.

The system of education, whether in social work or other disciplines, reflects and responds to the demands of the dominant culture's values and needs. The Council on Social Work Education (CSWE) stated that the social work profession was "guided by a person-in-environment perspective and respect for human diversity" and that "the profession works to effect social and economic justice worldwide" (CSWE, 2001, Educational Policy Standards, Preamble, paragraph one).

Several authors have stated that social work has failed to accomplish these educational goals and has lost the focus of social work's original mission: to fight for the poor and oppressed (Specht and Courtney, 1997; Gil, 1998). Gil (1998) wrote that "schools of social work prepare their students usually for practice in accordance with the status quo" and these institutions are "important components of oppressive and unjust societies" (p. 113). Freire (1970) explained the dominant culture's education structure through use of the analogy of the "banking system." The "banking system" involved a teacher (expert) who instilled (deposited) the relevant information into the student (learner) who was a passive receiver (an account) (Freire, 1970; hooks [sic], 1994). Freire (1970) and hooks [sic] (1994) described how this educational banking system treated students (and thereby clients) as objects, rather than active subjects in the education process. Current education standards foster this hierarchical model where students are trained to be experts in response to clients' social service needs.

Students need to become active participants in their education and institutions, and teachers need to relinquish some power and control to allow students more responsibility. Adrienne Rich (1977) called for students to realize that "you cannot afford to think of being here to receive an education; you will do much better to think of yourselves as being here to claim one" (p. 231). Several authors have written about the necessity of education, and social work education in particular, to operate from the perspective of the "student as an active participant," "student-centered," "subject-centered," or "student empowerment process of education" (Freire, 1970; hooks [sic], 1994; Gil, 1998; Palmer, 1998; Krishnamurti, 1953; Brookfield, 1987; Shor, 1998).

Students bring valuable life experience and knowledge to the classroom and this knowledge needs to be utilized and valued (Palmer, 1998; hooks [sic], 1994). Students need to be active and claim their voices and the cocreation of their education to make it more meaningful and relevant to their lives and work (Freire, 1970). Many students come to their education with a vital desire to connect, build relationships, and create community. Shor (1998) discussed the many ways that the student experience provides much of the grist for dialogue and learning. Social work education needs to begin with student experience and knowledge (like practice with the client), and from there the teacher can facilitate and enrich the process.

Although teachers are not the sole bestower of knowledge, their presence and knowledge are essential in the education process. Shor (1998) discussed how teachers draw out, enhance, facilitate, model, challenge, and support students in their learning. Similarily, Gil (1998) viewed the professor's role as that of "facilitator, advisor, resource, and nonauthoritarian, critical assistant, rather than 'expert,' authority, and judge" (p. 114). Gil (1998) believed that teachers need to "surrender to students [the] responsibility for their studies by eliminating teacher-set requirements and assignments, and by encouraging students to set these themselves" (p. 113).

Teachers help guide learning through "dialogical explorations" or "dialectical discussion," thereby involving students more fully in the process of education (Gil, 1998; Freire, 1970). Teachers not only facilitate the process of others' education but are in an "engaged pedagogy" or "liberatory pedagogy" as active learners themselves (hooks [sic], 1994). In this way, both teachers and students are teachers and learners. Both are active in the use and development of their self-knowledge and ability. Through this process teachers and students create a "cointentional education" (Freire, 1970).

Social group work or group-centered philosophies fit well with social work education. Group work has a rich history in the field of social work. In describing the movement of American group work, Alcorn, Epstein, and Rasheed (2001) reported that "group work was more than learning about methods; it was a lived experience about things like affiliation, learning community, experiential learning, less hierarchical ways of relating, and focusing on strengths" (pp. 1-2). The education of social workers today should indeed reflect its powerful history.

According to Parsons (1991), clients are empowered through their involvement in education groups, social action groups, and self-help groups. These groups "provide the opportunity for dialogue necessary for the development of critical thinking, knowledge and skill building, validation and support" (p. 13). One innovative social work program (Alcorn, Epstein, and Rasheed, 2001) seeks to integrate these ideas through the use of the group-centered perspective. Students and teachers at George Williams College are enhancing their "learning community" and achieving "less hierarchical ways of relating" by using the group-centered perspective. Through the use of this perspective, the teacher is no longer seen as a "giver of knowledge" and traditional student and teacher roles are challenged. Through collaborative learning the focus of education is on "critical thinking, reflexive learning and praxis-reflection, action, and reflection" (Alcorn, Epstein, and Rasheed, 2001, p. 16). The parallel process between teacher and student and practitioner and client, when viewed from a radical perspective, reveals that one challenge and strength in an emphasis on collaboration is "making friends with ambiguity and tolerating heightened contradictions that lead to more meaningful understandings" (Alcorn, Epstein, and Rasheed, 2001, p. 18).

The works of several authors who have written about how innovative and liberating education happens serve as a beginning point from which social work education can ask questions and be shaped. Freire (1970), hooks [sic] (1994), and Palmer (1998) placed emphasis on education as a "revolutionary" and "liberating" experience because it involved both student and teacher participation in the process of education. Freire (1970) and hooks [sic] (1994) proposed that education should be a liberating process for teachers and students instead of a static one-way exchange of knowledge. In this process, students become cocreators in their education and the classroom becomes an exciting and engaging place to learn (Freire, 1970; hooks [*sic*], 1994).

Lindeman (1926) believed that "all genuine education will keep doing and thinking together" and that "experience is the adult learner's living textbook" (as cited in Brookfield, 1987, p. 7). Revolutionary education moves students from an intellectual to a visceral understanding of life and its challenges, grounding knowledge and action in lived experience. Freire (1970) believed that for this revolutionary change to occur, people in their natural settings must come together to discuss ideas and the social and political impacts of institutions on their lives, and this interaction would lead to social transformation. This change will happen only if those who are impacted by an institution take action on their own behalf.

HISTORY OF THE RADICAL SOCIAL WORK STUDENT GROUP

The Radical Social Work Student Group (RSWSG) was formed January 2000. The idea for the group emerged from studying social group work and the settlement house movements of the early twentieth century during a history and philosophy of social work course. The founder of RSWSG, Stacy Husebo, was moved by the values and actions espoused by these early pioneers of a collective vision of caring for one another and joining together to share resources and build community. After studying the life of Jane Addams, Husebo brought together a group of seven students who possessed similar ideals to meet monthly to dialogue about ideas and paths of action that could be brought to the School of Social Work at the College of Saint Catherine and the University of Saint Thomas to enrich the education experience. The following vision statement was established to define the purpose of the group:

> We are a group of students committed to authenticity in our education and lives. We create dialogue and debate issues that challenge the status quo. We establish collaborative relationships with students, faculty and the broader community to become more deliberate about creating social transformation.

The group used the word *radical,* meaning that which proceeds from the root, the origin, or the essence. The ideals of the settlement house movement established the root or essence of the mission of the social work profession. For this reason, the student group found the word *radical* to be a fitting name for the group.

The RSWSG was an open group that met monthly to dialogue about issues that impact social work education in an effort to create social action to increase learning, impact social justice, and establish deeper and authentic relationships with students, faculty, and community members. A faculty liaison from the School of Social Work was selected by students. The faculty liaison offered additional information about radical social work ideals and connected the group to resources that enhanced members' understanding of radical ideas and practice.

STUDENT-FACULTY FORUM

After having met together for close to a year, the RSWSG decided that one way to create more intentional dialogue between students and faculty would be to plan and facilitate a group meeting. This dialogue event was labeled a student-faculty forum. The planning and execution of the forum reflected Kurland and Salmon's (1998) pregroup planning model (for use when group composition is not predetermined). According to this pregroup planning model, the need within the agency context defines the purpose, which in turn impacts the group composition, pregroup contact, as well as structure and content of the group.

As a group of students planning the forum, the *need* included having a voice in our education, conveying to the faculty our ability to educate and mobilize ourselves, as well as the need to build more authentic relationships with faculty. The *purpose* of the forum was to diminish traditional student and faculty power dynamics and build collaborative, authentic relationships based on shared learning. The RSWSG chose education as the student-faculty forum topic. The group determined that the purpose could be achieved by planning the content of the group around carefully designed questions and quotes from noted authors of education. As the need and purpose became clear, the faculty and administration at the School of Social Work *(the agency context)* encouraged the RSWSG to facilitate the student-faculty forum.

During two RSWSG planning meetings, group composition, pre-group contact, structure and content of the forum were discussed. The precise *group composition* was unknown, since it was unclear how many students and faculty would attend the forum. The RSWSG was mindful of the potential for the forum to be a "students versus the faculty" environment rather than a collaborative experience and worked to make the forum welcoming to everyone.

The *pregroup contact* involved members of the RSWSG personally inviting and mailing invitations to the forum to all students and faculty in the School of Social Work. The *structure* of the group would be a one-time meeting on January 25, 2001, with the possibility of future forums depending on the interest of students and faculty. The forum was scheduled for two hours in a classroom at the University of Saint Thomas. A welcoming environment was created by placing books about education by authors such as Paulo Freire, Adrienne Rich, J. Krishnamurti, bell hooks [*sic*], and Jonathan Kozol on a decorated table, having lighted candles, and posting inspirational quotes around the room.

The *content* of the group was determined by the purpose. To achieve the purpose of the forum and model collaboration, members of the RSWSG worked together to facilitate the group. Students introduced the RSWSG vision statement, clarified the purpose of the group, facilitated ground rule discussion, and answered questions. The large group was divided into two small groups, evenly dispersing the ten students, ten faculty, and two librarians. Students read quotes to the two small groups and then posed questions. After each question was posed, there was approximately fifteen minutes of small-group discussion. The last question was posed to the large group for a closing discussion.

PROGRAM EVALUATION

There were twenty-two participants in the forum: ten faculty, ten students, and two librarians. Fifteen participants completed a program evaluation. Four of the questions had a Likert scale ranging from 1 (strongly disagree) to 5 (strongly agree) and an area for comments. There were three open-ended questions.

All four of the Likert scale questions had a negatively skewed distribution (see Table 8.1 for frequency distributions). Fifteen (100 percent) respondents agreed that they had had an opportunity to speak and be heard at the forum. Twelve (80 percent) respondents agreed that the quotes had helped them to look at education in a different way. Fourteen (93 percent) respondents agreed that collaborative relationships between students and faculty had been developed at the forum. All respondents agreed that they would be interested in other forums.

Content analysis of the evaluations revealed the following five themes regarding what respondents liked about the forum: (1) students were active shapers in creating the forum, (2) authentic dialogue between teachers and students occurred, (3) collaborative relationships were initiated, which decreased hierarchical relationships, (4) teachers were learners and students were teachers, and (5) the learning was exciting and engaging because authentic stories and experiences were shared.

TABLE 8.1. Likert Scale Questions and Response Distributions

Question	Response Type	Response Distribution (%)	N
Did you have an opportunity to speak and be heard to-day?	4	20	3
	5	80	12
Did the quotes help you to look at education in a different way?	2	7	1
	3	13	2
	4	40	6
	5	40	6
Were collaborative relationships developed between students and faculty today?	3	7	1
	4	40	6
	5	53	8
Would you be interested in other forums?	5	100	14

Note: 1 = strongly disagree; 2 = disagree; 3 = neutral; 4 = agree; 5 = strongly agree.

DISCUSSION AND IMPLICATIONS

The first theme, that students were active shapers in creating the forum, was apparent by students planning, leading, and organizing the forum. This was done in an effort to claim the pieces of their education that they felt were missing. As students voiced their concerns and ideas about education, the faculty entered into the perspectives of the students. Faculty could let go of the expectation to be the experts and do all the teaching.

The second theme of authentic dialogue between teachers and students demonstrated how stimulating discussion bridged experiences between students and faculty. The third theme, that collaborative relationships were initiated, occurred by bringing faculty and students together in an informal manner to dialogue about experiences in education. Through this collaborative process, hierarchies and boundaries were dissolved, thus moving the discussion from an intellectual level to one grounded in the lived experience.

The fourth theme, that teachers were learners and students were teachers, was connected to the fifth theme, that learning was exciting and engaging because authentic stories and experiences were shared. Students and teachers gained a greater picture of education—a picture beyond their own experience and understanding of education. Students benefited by hearing how the teachers experienced their education, and teachers benefited by hearing how students experienced their education. The expectation of the professor to challenge students to think critically and the responsibility of students to be active and own their education was discussed.

Many comments made in the group discussion reflected these themes. Teaching and learning were described as creative, intuitive, an alive feeling, challenging, and passionate. The engaging learning experience was described as "repotting plants": The teacher challenged the student to learn and grow. As the student grew, the teacher challenged the student to go to the next level, to "repot." The paradox of being teachers and learners at the same time and the tension between teaching and letting go were discussed. Faculty and students were willing to dialogue, to exchange thoughts, beliefs, experiences, and ideas. The opportunity to be on the "same level" discussing education was appreciated by participants.

The student-initiated forum with faculty is one avenue for promoting restorative education. Institutions promoting student-led groups is another. For the experience to be effective, however, students need to take the initiative to challenge the status quo professor-student power differential. By the same token, teachers need to be receptive and supportive of student initiatives without being so involved that they take over the responsibility of collaborative efforts. Ironically, as institutions seek to empower students, or at least take that stance, students and communities do not always seize the opportunity. Moreover, there is a danger in institutionalizing student and community efforts. Co-opting such initiatives may create harmony at the loss of individual and communal diversity. Finding collaborative ventures where students and teachers are challenged to reveal their true colors is a difficult and complex task. It's arguably the most important task, as well.

Respondents indicated four ways to improve the forum: (1) increase attendance (of both students and faculty), (2) invite community members, (3) use separate rooms for break-out discussion, and (4) use fewer questions. In response to the question "What questions still need to be asked in regards to this topic?" respondents asked questions about where to go from here, how to continue the dialogue, and the implications for the classroom and course development. Topics suggested for future forums included how to nurture the qualities of passion, vision, and community in our program; the use of grades and evaluation; the future of social work; creating a safe environment in the classroom; and privilege in education.

The overwhelming positive responses from students and faculty regarding the forum experience indicate that more forums are welcome and perhaps needed. The forums could grow to include community members as well as student and faculty from other schools. Today, more than ever, social work needs to engage itself in activities such as the student-faculty forum. The benefits of restorative education and the community it generates and sustains are numerous. Students are enthused and empowered, develop a sense of competence, and are presented with the challenge of making a commitment to their education beyond the scope of "getting a degree." Faculty are also enthused and empowered, strengthen their competence, and are presented with the opportunity to develop a new vision of their students and make a commitment to them beyond the classroom. When social work education focuses on collaboration, community building, and looking outside its borders, it restores education to its proper place.

REFERENCES

Alcorn, S., Epstein, M., and Rasheed, M. (2001). The group-centered perspective: An ideology that found its home. Unpublished manuscript, George Williams College of Aurora University, Aurora, Illinois.

Brookfield, S. (1987). *Developing critical thinkers: Challenging adults to explore alternative ways of thinking and acting*. San Francisco: Jossey-Bass.

Council on Social Work Education, Inc. (CSWE) (2001). Educational Policy and Accreditation Standards. Retrieved from the Internet, August 27, 2001: <http://www.cswe.org/accreditation/EPAS/EPAS_start.htm>.

Cowger, C. (1994). Assessing client strengths: Clinical assessment for client empowerment. *Social Work, 39*(3): 262-268.

Freire, P. (1970). *Pedagogy of the oppressed*. New York: The Continuum Publishing Corporation.

Gil, D. (1998). *Confronting injustice and oppression: Concepts and strategies for social workers*. New York: Columbia University Press.

Gutiérrez, L. (1990). Working with women of color: An empowerment perspective. *Social Work,* March: 149-153.

hooks, b. [*sic*] (1994). *Teaching to transgress: Education as the practice of freedom*. New York: Routledge.

Kozol, J. (1981). *On being a teacher: RRR + values*. New York: Continuum.

Krishnamurti, J. (1953). *Education and the significance of life*. San Francisco: HarperCollins Publishers.

Krishnamurti, J. (1964). *Think on these things* (Ed. D. Rajagopal). New York: Harper & Row.

Kurland, R. and Salmon, R. (1998). *Teaching a methods course in social work with groups*. Alexandria, VA: Council on Social Work Education.

Palmer, P. (1998). *The courage to teach: Exploring the inner landscape of a teacher's life*. San Francisco: Jossey-Bass.

Parsons, R. (1991). Empowerment: Purpose and practice principle in social work. *Social Work with Groups,* 14(2): 7-21.

Rich, A. (1979). *On lies, secrets and silence: Selected prose 1966-1978*. New York: W.W. Norton and Co.

Shor, I. (1998). *Empowering education: Critical teaching for social change*. Chicago: University of Chicago Press.

Specht, H. and Courtney, M. (1997). *Unfaithful angels: How social work has abandoned its mission*. New York: Simon & Schuster.

Chapter 9

Group Simulation Projects: Teaching Group Work Skills in a Distance-Learning Classroom

Lonnie R. Helton
Edith M. Anderson

INTRODUCTION

Distance learning in higher education has become increasingly more prevalent within the last decade, and social work education has been an integral part of this innovation. An expanding body of literature points to the effectiveness of distance-learning classes and programs in social work education. In both urban and rural areas, distance learning programs have been developed in schools of social work for diverse reasons, such as cost-effectiveness, maximization of faculty resources, collaborative networking, information sharing, and continuing education.

Many studies emphasize the importance of the social context for teaching and learning, an important variable in understanding the differences between traditional and distance-learning classroom environments (Swartz and Biggs, 1999; Carnevale, 2000; Freddolino and Sutherland, 2000). Some have concentrated on student satisfaction with the distance-learning format and overall learning (Petracchi and Patchner, 2000). Moreover, several research studies on social work education using a variety of distance-learning approaches suggest that distance-learning course outcomes are fairly comparable with learning outcomes in traditional classroom settings (Klesius, Holman, and Thompson, 1997; Haga and Heitkamp, 2000; Freddolino and Sutherland, 2000; Petracchi and Patchner, 2000). Huff (2000) discovered, for instance, that students in a distance-learning graduate policy class acquired critical-thinking skills comparable to those achieved in a traditional classroom. Still, other researchers have found that graduate social work students rate teaching methods lower for two-way interactive television classes than for live instruction (Kreuger and Stretch, 2000; Thyer, Gaudin, and Polk, 1997).

Professional social work educators are challenged not only by the effective delivery of content but also by classroom process issues, especially with the teaching of relationship or "people" skills in social work practice methods classes. Freddolino (1996) noted that a wide range of roles in distance education must be carefully evaluated and monitored in reference to the development and maintenance of student and faculty/staff relationships. Potts and Hagan (2000) explored the use of systems theory in developing and evaluating distance education. Social work professionals have begun to explore the many avenues for group work provided by computer-based and distance-learning technology, such as e-mail, chat rooms, computer conferencing, and support groups (Bowman and Bowman, 1998).

The authors of this chapter describe the various methods and processes involved in teaching group work to a class of graduate social work students enrolled in a joint master of social work program using a distance-learning format. The universities are located approximately thirty-five miles apart in two adjoining metropolitan areas within northeastern Ohio.

METHODS OF TEACHING GROUP WORK VIA DISTANCE LEARNING

The authors have utilized a range of approaches to bring the students at the two distance-learning sites together as a working group. The language used to address the students suggests that the two sites have formed as one group for a cohesive "we" group experience. The students are encouraged to share e-mail addresses and many quickly begin to dialogue outside of class, both by e-mail and by using a Listserv, where students can post messages and share information about class work, student meetings, and other activities of interest on their respective campuses.

The Group Experience Project was developed with the goal of creating stronger relationships and group cohesion in a distance-learning setting. This project was implemented over an eight-week time frame and included all students in Advanced Practice with Small Systems II. For their Group Experience Project, students selected a theoretical framework, such as task-centered practice, reality therapy, or cognitive-behavioral therapy, and were asked to compare and contrast their group experiences with students in similar groups at the other site, as other students listened to and responded to their dialogue. This across-site sharing motivated students to offer additional ideas and suggestions via e-mail, faxes, and telephone calls. Such sharing helped to bond the class together as one group.

As a demonstration of how the group cohesion was solidified, the students got together at the end of the group work experience for a class project presentation and potluck supper, which gave them another opportunity to interact both formally and informally. This coming together exemplified the ritual of termination, as well, for the students then moved on to other course content for the rest of the semester. The authors also noted an increase in personal sharing among students overall once the group project experience occurred. The instructors also visited the alternate site a minimum of four times per semester, which strengthened their relationship even more with the distance-learning students, and provided an opportunity to encourage dialogue from a different perspective. Also, being in the presence of the students at the other site seemed to serve as a catalyst for further group sharing and cohesion within the larger group (i.e., the class as a whole). When at the distant site, the instructor exhibited a different presence with those students. This dynamic enhanced the engagement and processing of classroom content on group work.

In addition, the students function as one group across the two sites in that they continually interact with one another verbally and nonverbally to express their learning and application of theoretical frameworks of social group work. As they entered their Group Experience Project, they were expected to follow principles of group dynamics and group process that they had learned during the weekly lecture and discussion components of the class. The Group Experience Projects bring new information and insights concerning their application of the didactic content on groups covered in class. One might say that these subgroups function within the context of a naturally formed group.

Textbooks used for this graduate group work class were *An Introduction to Group Work Practice* (Fourth Edition) by R. W. Toseland

and R. F. Rivas (2001) and *Theory and Practice of Group Counseling* (Fifth Edition) by G. Corey (2000). The Toseland and Rivas (2001) textbook was used to cover broad group work dynamics and perspectives, whereas the Corey (2000) textbook was used to assist students in developing a specific theoretical framework for their group, which they utilized in leading the group, understanding group process, and documenting weekly meetings. The authors lectured on group dynamics, such as developmental stages, Bales' group process analysis (Bales, 1950), group roles, assessment, leadership styles, communication, and power.

CREATING AN EXPERIENTIAL LEARNING ENVIRONMENT BASED ON GROUP WORK PRINCIPLES

Structuring the classroom environment into the Group Experience Projects fostered an active learning experience and engaged students in a dynamic learning process. Many students who had not participated in groups previously were apprehensive. However, as they began to participate actively in their groups, they became aware of how social work with small groups impacts the change process, i.e., the steps involved in attaining the intended goals. Students were able to greatly expand their knowledge, enhance their skills, and advance their appreciation of the value of utilizing the group work process for helping client systems to develop and maintain adaptive functioning. As the students participated in their groups, they became better able to conceptualize that a major purpose of social group work is to facilitate the growth and development of its individual members. This became clearer to them as they worked together in their own groups and lived through the stages of group development.

The unique learning experience encompassed a small group (the Group Experience Project) functioning within a group (the class). Group process, group dynamics, and group interaction were quite revealing to all of us. The lecture and discussion in the class are designed to cover cognitive aspects of group work, such as Tuckman's and Bales' models of group development, problem solving and decision making, communication patterns, and group leadership. During this portion of the class, it became apparent that the students' bonding in their small groups carried over into the class. Small-group members were protective of the ideas and behaviors that were exhibited by a group member. Emphases were placed on skills and affective development in the small groups. Small-group members experienced the effect of Tuckman's developmental stages of forming, storming, norming, performing, and adjourning (Tuckman and Jensen, 1977). As students determined the type of group they wanted to become, as well as the theoretical model to be used, they experienced all of the five stages of group development. They also saw to a lesser degree this process in the larger group as the class functioned in a problem-solving and decision-making process.

The groups continued to seek an equilibrium between task and maintenance roles, to build effective relationships among group members, as described by Robert F. Bales (1950). A strong sense of mutual aid was effectively developed among group members as they attended to the emotional expressions of one another and the task-oriented needs of the group. Different group members seemed to have accepted one of these roles without anyone assigning them to a role. Rather, their role enactment was a natural extension of their personality. Both Tuckman and Jensen's sequential-stage perspective and Bales' recurring-phase perspective were useful in the students' understanding of group development.

As the groups entered the middle phase of development, they experienced the process of problem solving and decision making. The group interaction was frequently conflictual. However, they were able to "take care" of one another as they accomplished the group tasks. Naturally, there was a flow of positive and negative energy directed toward different group members. This was not constantly pointed toward a single member and did not take the form of a personal attack.

The group interaction, evidenced through their verbal and nonverbal communication patterns, was discussed in their biweekly journals and also depicted in their sociograms. While efforts were made to maintain group cohesion, relationship preferences were exhibited. The groups learned how to problem-solve by developing effective communication skills. They also experienced that the quality of the group's decision making directly relates to the group process. Through the small-group process, students' consciousness-raising regarding the impact of effective leadership and group facilitation was very significant. They learned the leader's roles and responsibilities from group formation to group termination. They became consciously aware of the importance of each individual's needs being met through the group process.

The lecture and discussions focused on utilizing the content from the Group Experience Projects to exemplify the theoretical and philosophical underpinnings of social work practice with groups. The students became aware that working with groups is similar to working with individuals, families, and communities. The same processes apply to all forms of social work practice, such as engagement, assessment, planning, intervention, termination, evaluation, and follow-up.

SUMMARY AND DISCUSSION OF IMPLICATIONS FOR GROUP WORK PRACTICE

The authors strongly believe that group work can be taught effectively in a distance-learning environment. Students have already become aware of the importance of sharing and participating in various assignments across the two distance-learning sites in other courses, and they have had opportunities to forge relationships with one another. The authors, in teaching group work, attempt to build on the students' willingness to engage in strategies that will bring the two subgroups of students within the class closer together as they study group dynamics and group process. The Group Experience Project gave students an opportunity to be part of a group and experience the roles of leader and participant. For some, it was their first opportunity to assume and practice a leadership role within a group. When the students converged at one site to present an analysis of their group project, this was a culminating experience for both students and faculty.

The authors will continue to use the methods described as well as other techniques that are likely to enhance across-site communication and bonding. The use of space and time, as well as "social presence," will remain challenges for any distance-learning environment. However, the instructors teaching this course must be forever mindful of the need for social work students to build strong interpersonal skills in preparation for work across multiple fields of practice. Although distance-learning classrooms make the teaching of group work and social work practice skills more challenging, the format offers new avenues for use of self, communication strategies, creativity, and critical analysis.

REFERENCES

Bales, R. F. (1950). A set of categories for the analysis of small group interaction. *American Sociological Review,* 15, 257-263.

Bowman, R. L. and Bowman, V. E. (1998). Life on the electronic frontier: The application of technology to group work. *Journal for Specialist in Group Work,* 23(4), 428-445.

Carnevale, D. (2000). A study produces a list of 24 benchmarks for quality distance education. *The Chronicle of Higher Education,* 46(31), A45.

Corey, G. (2000). *Theory and Practice of Group Counseling,* Fifth Edition. Belmont, CA: Brooks/Cole.

Freddolino, P. P. (1996). The importance of relationships for a quality learning environment in interactive TV classrooms. *Journal of Education for Business,* 71 (March/April), 205-208.

Freddolino, P. P. and Sutherland, C. A. (2000). Assessing the comparability of classroom environments in graduate social work education delivered via interactive instructional television. *Journal of Social Work Education,* 36(1), 115-129.

Haga, M. and Heitkamp, T. (2000). Bringing social work education to the prairie. *Journal of Social Work Education,* 36(2), 309-324.

Huff, M. T. (2000). A comparison of live instruction versus interactive television for teaching MSW students critical thinking skills. *Research on Social Work Practice,* 10(4), 400-416.

Klesius, J. P., Holman, S. P., and Thompson, T. (1997). Distance education compared to traditional instruction: The students' view. *International Journal of Instructional Media,* 24(3), 207-220.

Kreuger, L. W. and Stretch, J. J. (2000). How hypermodern technology in social work education bites back. *Journal of Social Work Education,* 36(1), 103-114.

Petracchi, H. (2000). Distance education: What do students tell us? *Research on Social Work Practice,* 10(3), 362-376.

Petracchi, H. and Patchner, M. A. (2000). Social work students and their learning environment: A comparison of interactive television, face-to-face instruction, and the traditional classroom. *Journal of Social Work Education,* 36(2), 335-346.

Potts, M. K. and Hagan, C. B. (2000). Going the distance: Using systems theory to design, implement, and evaluate a distance education program. *Journal of Social Work Education,* 36(1), 131-145.

Swartz, J. D. and Biggs, B. (1999). Technology, time, and space or what does it mean to be present? A study of the culture of a distance education class. *Journal of Educational Computing Research,* 20(1), 71-85.

Thyer, B. A., Gaudin, J., and Polk, G. (1997). Distance learning in social work education: A preliminary evaluation. *Journal of Social Work Education,* 33 (Spring/Summer), 363-367.

Toseland, R. W. and Rivas, R. F. (2001). *An Introduction to Group Work Practice,* Fourth Edition. Boston: Allyn and Bacon.

Tuckman, B. W. and Jensen, M. A. (1977). Stages of small group development revisited. *Group and Organizational Studies,* 2, 419-427.

Chapter 10

A Group Seminar to Enhance Field Instructors' Supervisory Skills

Kathleen Holtz Deal

Field instructors play a highly significant role in training social work students for practice. New field instructors are generally socialized to their role through a group orientation workshop (Lacerte and Ray, 1991). Beyond socialization, however, the needs of beginning supervisors are quite complex, since the process of learning to become an effective supervisor involves developing skills and abilities that differ from those the new supervisor developed as a practitioner (Stoltenberg, McNeill, and Delworth, 1998). With some exceptions (see, e.g., Fishbein and Glassman, 1991; Rogers and McDonald, 1992), field instructors are infrequently offered additional education or guidance beyond orientation, despite wide recognition that further training and support of field instructors is needed, particularly in exposure to theories of learning (Raskin, 1994). Because field instructors share many common experiences and needs, an interactive group seminar can offer a supportive environment for field instructors to expand their supervisory skills, thus furthering their development as educators and supervisors.

The purpose of this chapter is to describe and critique a twelve-hour, four-session group seminar for experienced MSW field instructors conducted in a school of social work in the mid-Atlantic United States. The chapter focuses on the seminar's educational content, membership, purpose, and activities. An evaluation of the group seminar regarding activities chosen, the leader's interventions, group purpose, and the development of group cohesion suggest recommendations for future seminars.

THE GROUP SEMINAR

Organizational Setting

Although the University of Maryland School of Social Work at Baltimore has consistently offered an introductory orientation for new field instructors, advanced or ongoing training has not been available through the Office of Field Instruction. Field instructor contacts concerning the individual learning needs and performance of students in the field were primarily through the field liaison. The Office of Field Instruction, however, targeted ongoing field instructor education as a goal. So when a faculty member developed an educational model for field instructor training, the field office decided to offer this model in a pilot seminar.

Group Members

Members were recruited through a letter sent to selected field agencies aimed at enlisting experienced field instructors. The letter explained the purpose of the seminar and offered continuing education units (CEUs) to participants. These efforts yielded eleven group members (eight female; three male). All were field instructors with two to fifteen years of experience working in agencies that served a wide range of client needs and ages. Some members knew others prior to beginning the seminar, including three members employed by the same agency. The group met in a seminar-style classroom at the school.

Leader

The faculty member who developed the training model led the group (see Deal, 2002, for a full explanation of the model). Although a current field liaison and former field instructor, she was relatively new to the school. The coordinator for field instruction performed a quasi-leadership role. He joined the seminar as a member with the purpose of learning the training model and assuming a leadership role in subsequent groups. He served a valuable role because of his years of experience at the school, knowledge of many seminar participants, and extensive knowledge of the field agencies.

Group Purpose

The group seminar was advertised as offering field instructors ways to expand their supervisory knowledge and skills through learning how to assess the normal stages of cognitive, affective, and behavioral development of MSW students and then tailor their supervision to fit their students' developmental learning needs. Although socioeducational groups are often formed to help members cope with a new role (Radin, 1985), the purpose of this group was to assist field instructors' development within their complex and demanding role.

Time

Meetings were held during the fall semester on four consecutive Friday mornings for three hours. Since CEUs were being offered, attendance was kept and members received credit only for the hours they actually attended. The seminar was held during work hours; therefore, agency emergencies sometimes affected participants' ability to attend or be on time.

Educational Content

The principal educational content of the seminar is a framework for the normative stages of MSW student development and guidelines for supervisory approaches recommended as most appropriate for each stage. The developmental models on which this framework is based (Friedman and Kaslow, 1986; Holman and Freed, 1987; Ralph, 1980; Saari, 1989; Stoltenberg, McNeill, and Delworth, 1998) describe typical cognitive, affective, and behavioral stages through which social work, counseling, and psychology trainees progress from entry into a graduate program to an independent level of practice. In general terms, these models describe students' cognitive progression from concrete, globalized, undifferentiated thinking to abstract, symbolic, and differentiated ways of understanding clients, situations, and theoretical concepts. Behaviorally, students gradually progress from rigid, stereotypic, action-oriented responses to flexible, individualized interventions that demonstrate an integration of theory and practice. Affectively, feelings of anxiety, self-consciousness, and dependence in beginning students change during the training process to feelings of increasing self-confidence and the desire for autonomy. These models further advocate ways that supervisors can enhance student development by attending to the particular characteristics and needs of each developmental stage. This educational content was primarily presented in the first two meetings of the seminar.

In addition, the content on students' developmental stages was used to develop a guide for field instructors to analyze student process recordings (see Deal, 2000, for a copy of the guide). This guide, which tracks eleven skills from beginning to advanced levels, was the focus for the third seminar meeting. The educational focus of the fourth meeting centered on specific techniques to help students progress along the developmental continuum. As with previous meetings, opportunities were provided for members to integrate learning and to share information about educational approaches they were trying with their students.

Activities

The educational content of the group seminar was presented in lecture discussion format to allow members to be exposed to and interact with the material. Handouts and slides supplemented the verbal presentation of material. Group exercises and discussion were used extensively to facilitate active participation. For example, group members were asked to generate a list of the characteristics of first- and second-year MSW students before being exposed to what the drafters of the developmental models had to say. An icebreaker exercise in which field instructors shared a funny or embarrassing thing they said or did as an MSW student elicited considerable affect, allowing field instructors to identify with the student role. Small-group discussions of case vignettes and student process recordings were followed by whole-group discussion on themes and common concerns. Homework assignments attempted to extend the group's purpose into the workplace environment. One assignment instructed members to write a process recording of one of their supervisory sessions; other group members then provided support and suggestions to that field instructor.

Group Process

A striking characteristic of the group was the degree of group support that quickly developed. Members appeared eager for opportunities to discuss common experiences and concerns with fellow field instructors. Their strong desire for contact suggested a sense of isolation in their role.

Although group support and cohesion predominated, the group developed some tension around two areas: group purpose and providing feedback to members. In terms of the group's purpose, this initially reflected the leader's views of what educational content would be useful and pertinent for field instructors. However, it is important for groups to accommodate members' goals in developing their purpose (Douglas, 2000; Kurland and Salmon, 1998), particularly in a socioeducational group where leaders and members have an egalitarian relationship (Radin, 1985). Therefore, at the first group meeting members were asked to share their needs and interests. Participants identified areas they wanted to see addressed in the seminar, including how to determine reasonable expectations for first- and second-year students, skills in handling problem students, and how to use process recordings as a supervision tool. Most of these areas of interest fit within the group purpose.

The needs of some members to resolve complex problems with individual students, however, could not be accommodated effectively given the group's purpose and time constraints. As is common in groups with a dual social and educational focus, tension occasionally developed when an individual member's needs to process and problem-solve a difficult situation threatened to dominate the group. An important task for the leader was refocusing the group when discussions of problem students or unresponsive administrators threatened to unbalance its socioeducational focus. One technique used was to help group members apply key concepts from the seminar's educational content to these supervisory problems, for example, understanding the student's developmental level and determining the best supervisory approach to use for that student. This approach helped the group shift from focusing on "What can I do with my problem student?" to "What are my student's specific developmental needs and how can I address them?" When successful, this activity both provided field instructors with concrete opportunities to apply their new learning and served to model how to apply theory to practice, an important supervisory behavior. When thinking developmentally was insufficient, field instructors were offered an opportunity to meet informally after the group with the leader or the coordinator of field instruction to discuss the problem. The coordinator of field instruction's extensive knowledge of the participants and the field instruction program made him a valuable resource for administrative and procedural concerns.

How to provide feedback to members who revealed the use of ineffective supervisory techniques was another area of tension for the group. Despite the fact that all members were experienced field instructors, participants had a wide range of supervisory skills. While one leadership task is to help more highly skilled members assist those with lower skills (Radin, 1985), this process demanded sensitivity in a group led by and composed of colleagues. Members generally offered feedback to one another in terms such as, "This is what I've found to work," thus avoiding direct confrontation. Tension emerged on rare occasions when a field instructor was unreceptive to members' suggestions, expressing comfort with their current supervisory approach.

EVALUATION

In a written evaluation, all members rated the educational content as either very or extremely useful to them. Several expressed the wish that they had had access to this information earlier in their careers as field instructors. All members agreed that the group seminar had met their expectations, with the majority indicating strong agreement. The activities rated as most effective included small-group exercises, handouts, and discussions with other field instructors. Many respondents included additional comments about how important the support, collegiality, and "collective wisdom" of other group seminar members were to them. Members generated many ideas for the future, including a desire for continued peer support in their role as field instructors, suggestions for the content of other seminars, and the establishment of a Field Advisory Committee to work with the Office of Field Instruction.

RECOMMENDATIONS

A minimum of four meetings are recommended to allow time for group members to begin to assimilate the seminar's educational content as well as to have some of their needs for support and affiliation met. An all-day seminar that included three-quarters of the educational material was subsequently tried as an alternative, but this format allowed fewer opportunities for members to integrate new learning or to form supportive relationships with other members. One of the key concepts of this seminar's educational content—that new learning is understood with greater complexity over time—argues for extending the time available for field instructors to contextualize and integrate new information with knowledge and skills they already possess.

Field instructors have generally been found to have an active learning style (Kruzich, Friesen, and Van Soest, 1986; Raschick, Maypole, and Day, 1998). Given this learning preference, participants in a similar seminar for field instructors could benefit from additional experiential methods. For example, Fishbein and Glassman (1991) made a video of one meeting of their field instructors' seminar that included members role-playing student–field instructor interactions. The video was then used for group critique and discussion of broad field instruction themes. For use in repeated seminars, leaders could make a prerecorded video of simulated role-plays involving various student–field instructor scenarios to stimulate discussion or role-playing by group members. Alternatively, field instructors could videotape an actual supervisory session (with the student's permission) and elicit feedback on their supervisory methods from the other members. This method might help seminar members provide more targeted feedback to one another. Using such methods may require lengthening the seminar; however, one or two follow-up meetings could address field instructors' needs for continued peer support.

Some of the most important learning in this seminar came from members assisting one another. Group leaders can play a role in this process by helping the group develop a trusting environment with norms that value giving and receiving feedback. Providing structured opportunities within the seminar where members can offer comments and suggestions based on role-plays or videotapes of supervisory conferences can give the kind of specific, targeted feedback that is most useful for growth.

Coleadership is recommended. Not only can coleaders bring complementary types of experiences to the seminar, but they can also share the roles of educator and facilitator. Seminar participants regarded CEUs as a significant benefit and a reward for their contributions to the field education program. From the school's perspective, CEUs reinforce the importance of advanced training.

Combining a clear, relevant educational focus with methodologies that provide frequent opportunities for active learning and peer interaction is recommended in designing similar field instructor seminars. Such group seminars can help support the need of field instructors to develop greater competence in their supervisory role.

REFERENCES

Deal, K. H. (2000). The usefulness of developmental stage models for clinical social work students: An exploratory study. *The Clinical Supervisor, 19*(1), 1-19.

Deal, K. H. (2002). Modifying field instructors' supervisory approach using stage models of student development. *Journal of Teaching in Social Work, 22*(3/4), 121-137.

Douglas, T. (2000). *Basic groupwork* (Second edition). London: Routledge.

Fishbein, H. and Glassman, U. (1991). The advanced seminar for field instructors: Content and process. In D. Schneck, B. Grossman, and U. Glassman (Eds.), *Field education in social work* (pp. 226-232). Dubuque, IA: Kendall/Hunt.

Friedman, D. and Kaslow, N. J. (1986). The development of professional identity in psychotherapists: Six stages in the supervision process. *The Clinical Supervisor, 4*, 29-49.

Holman, S. L. and Freed, P. (1987). Learning social work practice: A taxonomy. *The Clinical Supervisor, 5*(1), 3-21.

Kruzich, J. M., Friesen, B. J., and Van Soest, D. (1986). The assessment of student and faculty learning styles: Research and application. *Journal of Social Work Education, 22*, 22-30.

Kurland, R. and Salmon, R. (1998). Purpose: A misunderstood and misused keystone of group work practice. *Social Work with Groups, 21*(3), 5-17.

Lacerte, J. and Ray, J. (1991). Recognizing the educational contributions of field instructors. In D. Schneck, B. Grossman, and U. Glassman (Eds.), *Field education in social work* (pp. 217-225). Dubuque, IA: Kendall/Hunt.

Radin, N. (1985). Socioeducational groups. In M. Sundel, P. Glasser, R. Saari, and R. Vinter (Eds.), *Individual change through small groups* (Second edition) (pp. 101-112). New York: The Free Press.

Ralph, N. B. (1980). Learning psychotherapy: A developmental perspective. *Psychiatry, 43,* 243-250.

Raschick, M., Maypole, D. E., and Day, P. A. (1998). Improving field education through Kolb learning theory. *Journal of Social Work Education, 34*(1), 31-42.

Raskin, M. S. (1994). The Delphi student in field education revisited: Expert consensus on issues and research priorities. *Journal of Social Work Education, 30*(1), 75-89.

Rogers, G. and McDonald, P. L. (1992). Thinking critically: An approach to field instructor training. *Journal of Social Work Education, 28*(2), 166-177.

Saari, C. (1989). The process of learning in clinical social work. *Smith College Studies in Social Work, 60,* 35-49.

Stoltenberg, C. D., McNeill, B., and Delworth, U. (1998). *IDM Supervision: An integrated developmental model for supervising counselors and therapists.* San Francisco: Jossey-Bass.

PART IV:
GROUP WORKERS FACING NEW
AND UNPREDICTABLE SITUATIONS

Chapter 11

Yo no hablo Español: Facilitating a Group in Another Language

Patricia M. Merle

Many of the tasks of a facilitator—keeping the discussion on target, mediating, clarifying (AASWG, 1999)—need a common language in order to be performed. Can there be value in facilitating a group when there is no common language and in fact very dissimilar cultures? Last year I had the opportunity to explore these questions when my colleague and I, neither of whom speaks Spanish, were invited to give a workshop to a group of women in Mexico.

BACKGROUND

Anapra is one of many villages in the Chihuahua desert settled by people from the interior of Mexico who come to work in the *maquiladoras* (American and Japanese factories on the border). At the time of this writing, there was no running water, telephones, or paved roads (just tracks in the sand) in Anapra. Most of the 16,000 people live in houses made of wooden pallets and tarpaper.

Grupo Amistad is a group of six women who live in Anapra with their families and as volunteers oversee the work sponsored in the *colonia* by St. Mark's Church of Independence, Missouri. Some of their tasks include selecting families to receive tuition assistance and overseeing the purchase and distribution of books, school supplies, and uniforms to these families. They pay the tuition for 150 children and monitor their grades. They also distribute food and clothing and select needy families to have a house built for them by volunteers.

My colleague and I have gone to Anapra every year for the past seven years to visit the people and help out where needed. We have been continually amazed at the amount of communication that occurs without a common language (my high school Spanish gives me some vocabulary, but I cannot understand spoken Spanish). Knowing about our work with women in prison, the women asked us to give a workshop to Grupo Amistad because they feel the need to be nurtured themselves. We were surprised, since they are well aware of our lack of Spanish language, and only one of the women in the group speaks English. Two factors influenced us to agree: first, the ability we have had to develop relationships with one another in spite of the lack of a common language and, second, the lack of resources in Anapra for the women themselves to find nourishment. Without any idea of how we would overcome the language barrier, we agreed to offer a workshop the next time we came to Anapra.

ISSUES

When I began to design the workshop months before the trip, the first problem I encountered was that I had to find activities in which language was not the primary means of communication. I adapted three activities we have used in our work in which the participants draw symbols of their thoughts or needs and then discuss the content. Since art is a universal language, we could understand the symbols and would have some idea of the content of the women's work.

In our previous visits, Estela, who speaks English, had been the link between us and the other women. We considered using her as translator, but felt that it was not fair to her as a participant to have the duty of also translating. Our observation of the dynamics in the group in previous years had been that, as the leader, Estela would speak to and for the others. The other members would go along with whatever decisions she made since she had the power of being the only bilingual person in the group. We hoped that having Estela as an equal participant with the other women would help to equalize relationships. We wanted to give each woman an opportunity to use her own voice in the group, rather than depend on a translator.

Translation Issues

Because we would not be using a translator, we tried to anticipate what might occur in the group. First, I wrote out the activities of each session, the directions for the activities, and any explanations necessary. Then I wrote out the introductions and summaries of each session. Finally, my colleague and I brainstormed "what if" possibilities. What if someone interrupts? What if someone doesn't participate? What if . . . ? We wrote out a list of ten or so sentences we could use if any of these possibilities occurred.

Five bilingual volunteers spent many hours translating this material into Spanish. Two issues that became apparent were that I had no way to judge the quality of the translators' work, and I did not know whether their Spanish would be understandable to the women, since there are many differences in language and culture among Latino groups (Gutiérrez and Suarez, 1999; Weaver and Wodarski, 1996).

Once the translations were done and revised, I spent many hours reading them out loud, to increase the chances that I would be clear, fluent, and understandable. One translator helped me with pronunciation and deciding where to break up long sentences, since I knew that pausing in the wrong place could cause confusion.

Planning, preparing, and translating this workshop and trying to anticipate possible responses were the first indications that the differences in language would require enormous amounts of work and energy even before the actual workshop.

THE WORKSHOP MODEL

The workshop we offered at Anapra is based on workshops that we have been offering in correctional facilities for many years. The mission of Step by Step, a program founded by myself and a colleague ten years ago, is to help incarcerated women tell their stories and find in their stories the gifts and strengths that they possess so that they can then use these gifts and strengths to build new lives for themselves (Merle, 2000). Step by Step believes that, for oppressed women, it is much more helpful to come from a strengths-based perspective (Early and GlenMaye, 2000; Postmus, 2000; Saleeby, 1996, 1997, 2001) than a problem-focused one. This approach builds on what is right with people rather than what is wrong with people (Pollio, Mc-Donald, and North, 1996). Since "groups are natural vehicles for empowerment" (Breton, 1994, p. 30; also Parsons, 2001), this process of sharing stories in a group helps to bring forth each woman's gifts and strengths. It was this workshop model that we agreed to adapt for the women of Anapra.

Outline of the Anapra Workshop

The theme I chose for the workshop was "Let the Desert Rejoice" because, even with the lack of water, most families use wastewater to grow flowers in the sand. The first day I read the script, introducing the theme of the workshop, and then gave the ground rules (which we would normally have the group set, one of many difficulties of facilitating in an unknown language). These included the following:

1. Listen with respect when others are speaking. (Escuchen con respeto cuando otras están hablando.)
2. Do not comment on another's answer. She has a right to her opinion. (No juzguen las respuestas de otras. Ella tiene el derecho de opinar.)
3. Do not give advice. We have within ourselves our own answers. (No den consejo. Tenemos en nosotras mismas nuestras propias respuestas.)

After the ground rules and an icebreaker activity (more below about the difficulties of facilitating games in another language), the primary task of this first session was for the women to name their needs as a group. Each woman was invited to speak in turn and the needs named were listed on newsprint (by one of the women). Although there was a lot of shyness and resistance at first, this soon dissipated. By the end of the first session, all women were sharing, volunteering to talk, and seemingly enjoying the experience.

The second day the women were divided into two groups and invited to draw symbols of the needs named the day before. Then each team explained to the other team what they had drawn and what the meaning was of each symbol. With each activity in the workshop, every woman took turns to tell about her drawing or work. This was an opportunity to practice speaking for herself and the first step in proclaiming her own voice (Parsons, 2001).

The third day each woman drew flowers to represent the gifts or strengths of the other members of the group. When the flowers were drawn, we went around the group, asking each woman to choose one flower and name the gift or strength it represented for a particular woman. This process was repeated until each woman had named two gifts and strengths for each of the other women. After this was over, each woman was called on to name two gifts or strengths in herself. The flowers were then formed into a bouquet and pasted onto a poster board. The bouquet was hung on the wall as a visible symbol and reminder of the group's gifts and strengths.

On the fourth day they were each given some large puzzle pieces and were asked to draw on each one something that Grupo Amistad does in the *colonia*. Then they were given more puzzle pieces to draw what other groups who provide services in the *colonia* are doing. They taped all these pieces together and when the puzzle was turned over, it was a picture of a circle of people holding hands, surrounded by flowers. Then I asked them to look at all the activities being done in the *colonia,* by themselves and by others. "Many flowers are blooming in the desert, because of your work and the work of others. When we put all our efforts together, we form a circle of community and the desert will flower." ("Muchas flores están floreciendo in el desierto, como resultado de su servicio y el servicio de otros. Cuando nosotros ponemos todos nuestros esfuerzos juntos, formamos un circulo comunidad y el desierto florecerá.")

FACILITATION PROBLEMS

At times we became aware of issues that we could not deal with because we didn't have the words to change or challenge what was happening. In the first class, we asked the women what they saw as the needs of the group. Bertha, who volunteered to go first, said that she had two answers. Each woman followed her lead and gave two answers. The last person to speak was harder pressed to come up with original needs. We had not anticipated this problem and so did not have the words to say in Spanish, "Let's just say one now and we'll come back for a second round." We had to let the process continue.

Another example of misunderstanding was that the women had obviously made assumptions about the workshop and brought pencils and paper. The first night, every time we said something, they wrote it down. We didn't know how to say, "Put down your pencils and just listen now, we are going to play a game." When it came time for the name game, which depends on the challenge of each person remembering everyone else's name and adjective, the point was lost, since each woman wrote down everyone's name and adjective and then read it.

A more serious example of what we missed because of language was when the women listed strengths for one another for the bouquet. That evening we looked up all the strengths in our English-Spanish dictionary so that when we listed them on their certificates we would be sure they were spelled properly. We were unable to find *aporona,* which had been given for one woman. The next day we asked how to spell the word and found out that its meaning is "worries too much about everything." If we had understood the meaning at the time of the naming, we would have said, "That can sound judging. How do you see it as a strength in Olga?" We had had no idea that a negative word had been used, but even when we realized the problem the following day, not having the language to deal with the issue made it difficult to act. So we did not. To have begun to intervene and then not have the words to clarify and solve the situation might have made it worse.

CULTURE CLASH

We did not have to wait long to see two cultures clash. If our culture is based on power, while the Mexican culture is based on relationship (Poole, 1998; Weaver and Wodarski, 1996), we witnessed an illustration of this difference in the first session. In the activity for this class, we asked, "What do you see as the needs of the group to accomplish your tasks in the next year?" Our expectation was that they would list activities they could do as a group for the good of the *colonia:* build more houses, follow up on enrollment in school better, develop a form for keeping track of . . . , etc. As they listed their responses, I sat there in dismay as they said, *compartir, comprensión, hermandad, amistad, alegría, armonía, comunicación, sinceridad, amor,* and *unión* (sisterliness, friendship, happiness, harmony, communication, sincerity, love, and togetherness). I assumed that they had misunderstood the question. After they completed their list, I then asked the question again, adding the phrase "in the *colonia*" to refocus on the "correct" agenda (even though we had insisted in the beginning that there is no right or wrong). This time their responses were more in line with what we expected: to help people in the *colonia*, to serve and be more helpful, to have people learn how we can help.

In planning for the next session and reviewing their responses, I realized that I had made the assumption that we, as experts, knew best what the group needed (Breton, 1992; Breton, 1994; Gutiérrez and Suarez, 1999; Salzer, Rappaport, and Segre, 1999). As the group leader, I had assumed, as Rose (2000, p. 404) writes, the "power to name another person's experience." I learned from their responses what they personally need to keep the group serving and growing (Davis, 1995; Weaver and Wodarski, 1996). As insiders, they knew that the group had internal strains that needed to be worked out before they could focus on organization building (Staples, 2000). Because of this realization of how I had co-opted the agenda, I had to refocus our approach for session two to stay with their agenda instead of my own (Peled et al., 2000). I had made assumptions based on our own cultural beliefs of organizational strength and almost dismissed their cultural beliefs that relationship has priority over tasks.

BENEFITS

The women of Grupo Amistad had the experience in this workshop of having a voice, and this voice being heard and responded to (Gutiérrez and Suarez, 1999; Parsons, 2001). We saw several examples of behavior change as the workshop progressed. First, several women began moving the group along with humor and took ownership of the process we had modeled. Irene began saying "Un minuto" when the time for an activity was coming to an end. Second, most of the women began to see to it that everyone took turns. Estela would begin an activity and then give the marker to Mari to continue the task. Third, we "know" Mari as painfully shy and retiring, so it was with great pleasure that by the end of the workshop she volunteered to go first, reading with great pride and making everyone laugh with her sense of humor.

Fourth, the last night, when they were asked to draw what they do in the *colonia,* their drawings were intricate and detailed. They obviously were enjoying the drawing since they spent more and more time adding more and more details. Fifth, in the last session, we asked them to evaluate the workshop. By this time, we were so exhausted that without thinking, we tried to collect their evaluations without having them read them out loud first. They immediately protested, asking if we didn't want to hear them first. Sixth, when we asked for permission to use their work, their body language showed that they were thrilled to be asked. By this time we were absorbing their meanings by osmosis and so somehow we know that they are honored to think that their work might be used to help teach others that language does not have to stand in the way. "Tell them . . . ," they kept saying.

Because we are culturally trained to have less faith in the certainty of our intuition and our other senses (Stempler, 1992), we are reluctant to claim that the women benefited from this workshop. However, there were many indications that they did benefit. They came to every class and were on time. They fully participated, obviously laughed and enjoyed themselves, brought the kids if necessary so they could attend, and began to practice some of what we had taught them. They also asked us to return next year to do another workshop. They wrote in their evaluations that it was good to learn more about one another and to feel stronger bonds among them.

RELEVANCE

The women asked for a group process in which they could be energized for their volunteer work in the coming year. The focus of the workshop we designed was to help the women name their gifts and strengths and celebrate them, as well as to see their work as part of the larger picture of efforts in Anapra. Naming and celebrating their strengths and seeing themselves as part of a larger picture are two ways to nurture their work.

We did not know what they would name as their needs when we planned the workshop. The beauty of the strengths perspective is that it puts the responsibility on the group members to find their own solutions. They are not dependent on the "expert" for their answers. No matter what they had named as their needs, the workshop, with its emphasis on each woman having a voice, being listened to with respect, and not being judged, would have filled these needs by having them answer these questions: What are your needs? What are your gifts and strengths? What is the work that you are doing in the *colonia?*

For example, their most frequently expressed needs for the workshop were an increase in friendship, unity, and communication, responses we had not anticipated at all. Because the structure of the sessions called for each woman to participate equally, *communicación* among them was enhanced by hearing everyone's voice. Friendship *(amistad)* was strengthened by hearing and sharing one another's thoughts, dreams, and hopes. The *unión* of the group was enhanced as they shared their thoughts without judgment or advice giving.

At the end of the four sessions, we asked the women to evaluate the sessions and write down what was most helpful to them. Yolanda, as the newest member, said that she liked the first day because they learned to share more with one another. (El primer día porque nos enseño a conservenor más entre compañeras, y saber nuestras inquietudes, y poner en práctica en nuestras semejanzas que es el Rancho Anapra.) Estela, as group leader, chose the first drawing exercise because she sees the important things that, as Grupo Amistad, they need to nurture in order to keep going. She added that the most important thing was to come to the workshop and share as they did. (La de los cofres porque veo las más necesarias cosas que como Grupo Amistad necesitamos alimentor para seguir siempre adelante. Pero lo más importante fue el venir y convivir en el taller como lo hicimos esta semana. Gracias, Pat y Margy.)

Mari and Bertha both picked the bouquet exercise as their favorite, Mari because she liked the idea of her group and the other groups being represented by flowers in the desert, and Bertha because she enjoyed naming strengths and gifts for the other members of the group and because she now identifies herself as a flower growing in the desert. (Mari: Como mi grupo me gustó mucho el de las flores como representamos nuestro grupo como flores en el desierto y también los otros. Bertha: La que más me gustó fue el de las flores. Porque tubé la oportunidad de decirles a mis compañeras sus virtudes y sus fortalezas, y porque desde ese día me identifico con una flor. Y seré para siempre una flor que creció en el desierto.)

Irene chose the puzzle because it made her realize how much work is being done in the *colonia* by other groups and she had not realized this before. (A mi me ayudó la del rompecabeza. Porque me di cuenta de grupos que hay en la comunidad. Y yo no me daba cuenta. Gracias, Pati y Margarita.) Olga said she is glad to know that she and everyone in the group thinks the same way about the group and so they are all traveling on the same path. (El saber lo que pienso y pensamos de nuestro grupo todas porque así supe y me confortó el saber que todas vamos dirigidas hacía el mismo camino. La convivencia con todas.)

CONCLUSION

Schmitz (1998) took a group of social work students to Mexico for an educational experience of a third world country and the cultural privilege we enjoy in a developed nation. She wrote about the frustration of listening without being able to respond and the necessity of using all her senses to listen and communicate. We experienced similar frustrations and were often on edge because of the need to concentrate so totally with all our senses. We were aware that we had missed some of the dynamics in the group. However, judging by the mood in each session, the eagerness of each woman to participate, the evaluations, and the change in behavior over the four sessions, the intensity of the preparation and the toll on us as facilitators was worth it.

In our workshop, the women experienced everyone taking a turn and sharing a variety of tasks. They learned about their own and one another's creativity and the gifts and strengths of each woman in the group. Their work in small groups gave the opportunity for each woman to experience being a leader. The quiet ones were given the opportunity to speak and the vocal ones were encouraged to listen. The *rompacabeza* (the puzzle they put together in the last class) graphically illustrated for them the value and magnitude of their work as well as their connection with other groups. All of these experiences stretched them and gave them a bigger vision, as well as the opportunity to be affirmed and appreciated for the work they do.

As Saleebey (2001, p. 221) has written, "the work to be done, in the end, depends on the resources, reserves, and assets in and around the individual, family, or community." This workshop gave the women of Grupo Amistad an opportunity to recognize and acknowledge the gifts and strengths they bring, individually and as a group, to the work of the *colonia*. They experienced a model of group leadership where all voices are heard and everyone's gifts and strengths are acknowledged and acclaimed. It is now the work of the group (Stempler, 1992) to find a way to use these experiences to fill their needs for *amistad, unión,* and *comunicación.*

REFERENCES

AASWG (1999). *Standards for Social Work Practice with Groups.* Akron, OH: Association for the Advancement of Social Work with Groups, Inc.

Breton, M. (1992). Clinical social work: Who is being empowered? In D.F. Fike and B. Rittner (Eds.), *Working from Strengths: The Essence of Group Work.* Miami, FL: Center for Group Work Studies, pp. 81-86.

Breton, M. (1994). On the meaning of empowerment and empowerment-oriented social work practice. *Social Work with Groups,* 17(3), 23-37.

Davis, L.E. (1995). The crisis of diversity. In M.D. Feit, J.H. Ramey, J.S. Wodarski, and A.R. Mann (Eds.), *Capturing the Power of Diversity.* Binghamton, NY: The Haworth Press, pp. 47-57.

Early, T.J. and GlenMaye, L.F. (2000). Valuing families: Social work practice with families from a strengths perspective. *Social Work,* 45(20), 118-130.

Gutiérrez, L.M. and Suarez, Z. (1999). Empowerment with Latinas. In L.M. Gutiérrez and E.A. Lewis (Eds.), *Empowering Women of Color.* New York: Columbia University.

Merle, P.M. (2000). A narrative analysis of the meaning of the gifts and strengths of women in prison as expressed in their life stories. Unpublished dissertation. Columbia University School of Social Work, New York.

Parsons, R.J. (2001). Specific practice strategies for empowerment-based practice with women: A study of two groups. *Affilia,* 16(2), 159-179.

Peled, E., Eisikovits, Z., Enosh, G., and Winstok, Z. (2000). Choice and empowerment for battered women who stay: Toward a constructivist model. *Social Work,* 45(1), 9-25.

Pollio, D.E., McDonald, S.M., and North, C.S. (1996). Combining a strengths-based approach and feminist theory in group work with persons "on the streets." *Social Work with Groups,* 19(3/4), 5-20.

Poole, D.L. (1998). Politically correct or culturally competent? *Health and Social Work,* 23(3), 163-166.

Postmus, J.L. (2000). Analysis of the family violence option: A strengths perspective. *Affilia,* 15(2), 244-258.

Rose, S.M. (2000). Reflections on empowerment-based practice. *Social Work,* 45(5), 403-412.

Saleebey, D. (1996). The strengths perspective in social work practice: Extensions and cautions. *Social Work,* 41(3), 296-305.

Saleebey, D. (1997). *The Strengths Perspective in Social Work Practice.* White Plains, NY: Longman.

Saleebey, D. (2001). Practicing the strengths perspective: Everyday tools and resources. *Families in Society,* 82(3), 221-222.

Salzer, M.S., Rappaport, J., and Segre, L. (1999). Professional appraisal of professionally led and self-help groups. *American Journal of Orthopsychiatry,* 69, 536-540.

Schmitz, C.L. (1998). Tortillas and salt: Lessons across North America. *Reflections,* Spring, 21-32.

Staples, L.H. (2000). Insider/outsider upsides and downsides. *Social Work with Groups,* 23(2), 19-35.

Stempler, B.L. (1992). There are so many of them and only one of me: Developing and utilizing natural strengths in learning to lead mutual aid groups. In D.F. Fike and B. Rittner (Eds.), *Working from Strengths: The Essence of Group Work.* Miami, FL: Center for Group Work Studies, pp. 162-181.

Weaver, H.N. and Wodarski, J.S. (1996). Social work practice with Latinos. In D.F. Harrison, B.A. Thyer, and J.S. Wodarski (Eds.), *Cultural Diversity and Social Work Practice,* Second Edition. Springfield, IL: Charles C Thomas, pp. 52-86.

Chapter 12

"How Can I Talk About This Stuff?" Mutual Aid and Group Development in a Collectivity for Persons with Ulcerative Colitis

Catherine Coulthard
Joanne Sulman
Brenda O'Connor

I went to the group only four days after my surgery, when I was still in the hospital. I could actually see all these people who survived it, and it made me feel so much better to know that I'm not alone. I was in the process—just brand new—so that helped a lot.*

Looking at the "somewhat checkered history" of social group work in health settings, Thomas Carlton (1986) reminded us that groups are usually an add-on to caseloads that are already burdensome. Despite this daunting fact, over the past fifteen years the group work literature in health care has blossomed. A recent online search found dozens of examples of social work groups on a rich array of topics from single-session, waiting-room groups to trauma support and preadmission discharge planning. Parry (1980) suggests that one of the major purposes of groups in health settings is to help the mem-

The authors wish to acknowledge the unfailing, tangible support from the Inflammatory Bowel Disease Program and its team members, and the inspiration and dedication of Karen Witkowski, RN, BScN, ET; Pat Reed, MSW, RSW; and the members of the Pelvic Pouch Steering Committee.
*All quotes from group members and their spouses are from 2001.

bers feel as normal as possible within the constraints of their chronic condition or disability. One of the members of the group that we will describe in this article illustrates Parry's point:

> The group was mentioned to us while we were in the hospital as a great way to meet people in the same predicament and exchange good *healthy* information, and that's exactly what it's been.

The overall purpose of the paper is to look at the ways in which an education program for persons with ulcerative colitis transformed itself into a genuine mutual aid support system. The narratives of group members are a counterpoint to the text since they express, far more eloquently than the authors, the nature of the helping process in the Pelvic Pouch Support Group.

BACKGROUND OF THE GROUP PROGRAM

Origins of the Group

Several years ago, in a Canadian university teaching hospital, an outpatient collectivity called the Pelvic Pouch Support Group began at the urging of persons with ulcerative colitis and their families. One group member describes his initial feelings of confusion and isolation:

> When I was first diagnosed it was ignorance. . . . I honestly didn't know people could live without a colon. Once you leave the hospital you feel very, very vulnerable because there's not a soul out there—you're alone.

Ulcerative colitis, a form of inflammatory bowel disease (IBD), commonly strikes adolescents and young adults. The patients who were requesting a support group had undergone a series of major surgeries known as "the pelvic pouch procedure" that potentially would cure their disease and relieve their symptoms. Unfortunately, there are often sequelae of the surgeries that create ongoing problems. Thus, the dual indicators of patient need and the fact that no community support programs existed in Toronto for this population convinced hospital staff to sponsor the group.

Structure: This Group Is a Collectivity

As noted in the chapter title, the support group is in fact a loose-knit collectivity of patients, family members, and friends. According to Norma Lang (1987), a collectivity is "a limited social form structured in such a way that advancement to group is precluded." The Pelvic Pouch Support Group was developed on a psychoeducational model, with professional leadership from nursing and social work, and support from medicine, nutrition, and pharmacy. Staff assumed responsibility for all aspects of program planning and service delivery. This included the organization and facilitation of the meetings, the creation of a newsletter, and the management of a buddy program.

Since its inception, the collectivity has met once every two months for two hours, with a program consisting of guest speakers and a bit of time for networking. Persons with ulcerative colitis are often reluctant to talk to others about their bowel symptoms. As a member wryly notes, "It's hardly table talk." The collectivity created a safe environment for sharing experiences, struggles, and suggestions.

> It's funny because you can share a lot of stories and talk about a lot of things that you can't with everyday people. I think people [in the group] are very comfortable even with strangers to say very personal things.

Transitioning Leadership

Functionally, the Pelvic Pouch Support Group is an open system because of the continuous intake of new members (Schopler and Galinsky, 1995). To add to the complexity, the group has been through a number of changes in professional leadership, as some staff members have left and others have joined the program. Despite these shifts, the group maintained continuity through the structure and format of the meetings and the presence of at least one familiar staff face. Undeterred by the constant flux, a core group of members formed connections to one another, and their commitment to the support group acted as a stabilizing force during periods of transition.

Not surprisingly, a hospital climate of change and cutbacks discouraged an examination of options for group development, but with a reinfusion of both social workers and nurses two years ago, staff took the opportunity to evaluate the program.

Program Evaluation

The evaluation looked at the distance between the collectivity's historical manner of functioning and new goals that included enhanced mutual aid and peer leadership. Even though a core subgroup of members attended regularly, program and process had scant member input. As a loose-knit collectivity, the Pelvic Pouch Support Group mimicked the beginning stages of group life at each meeting. In other words, this was a laid-on mass program that had no hope of self-maintenance, and that's exactly what the fifteen to seventy people who attended meetings seemed to want.

One of the social work staff, a group worker, suggested the development of some of the collectivity's subsystems to increase member involvement in structure and process. This began an evolution of the collectivity toward a more autonomous format, with the following goals identified as group development initiatives: to strengthen mutual support networks, to empower indigenous leadership, to move from a psychoeducational model to a mutual aid/self-help model, and to alter the role of the professional from group leader to group worker, consultant, and provider of practical support.

Maturing groups have the ability to move through stages of development toward differentiation and autonomy as members connect, interact authentically, and provide mutual aid to one another in pursuit of common goals. The Pelvic Pouch Support Group, with its infrequent meetings and large numbers of people who sporadically attend those meetings, is not able to become a mature group. Nevertheless, staff believed that it was possible to restructure the collectivity's organization to enhance its helping qualities. The next step was an examination of the collectivity in the context of the literature on self-help groups, empowerment, mutual aid, membership, and the role of the professional.

LITERATURE REVIEW

Self-Help

> We're really like a user group. I was rather expecting problems, and also expected people to have similar problems. In talking with other people regarding solutions, this spreads solutions to other members of the group.

Wituk and colleagues (2000) describe self-help groups as being comprised of persons who share the same problem, who provide emotional support to one another, learn coping strategies, and help others while helping themselves. Schopler and Galinsky (1995) view support groups as open systems that are member centered. Coplon and Strull (1983) underscore the link between self-help and mutual aid. Kurtz and Powell (1987) note that "often the set of social relationships available to people in distress proves incapable of providing the necessary support" (p. 71), and they attribute some benefits of self-help groups "to new and strengthened relationships in a more adequate social network" (p. 70). Peer support offers something that professional intervention cannot, namely, the shared reality of similar personal experience: "I've been there." One group member described her need to talk to others who understood her distress:

> You don't want to remember the pain, the nights you didn't sleep and thought you would die in the bathroom—then it's like a release—you get to release how you felt when you meet in the group.

Empowerment

> When we first started coming, we were on the learning curve. Now we can help with the emotional side of "What am I going through?" and the life experience of it. (Spousal member)

Self-help, by definition, implies empowerment. Pernell (1986) first introduced the term to social group work: "Groups are a natural context for efforts toward empowerment . . . and group workers traditionally have the skills which are needed to help members make the most of opportunities" (p. 114). How do groups empower their members?

According to Parsons (1991), support groups "provide the opportunity for dialogue necessary for the development of critical thinking, knowledge and skill building, validation and support" (p. 13). Mutual aid or self-help groups have the opportunity to forge a network that not only provides support, motivation, and practical help for members but also gives them the chance to take leadership on issues of importance to them. As Breton (1994a) points out, "Mutual aid groups are ideal places for people to find and to learn to use their voices— necessary conditions for empowerment" (p. 32). Members of mutual aid groups engage in authentic collective decision making and experience their own expertise in helping others deal with common concerns. They can also initiate social action in their communities (Breton, 1995). Fagan and Stevenson (1995), in their discussion of a self-help parenting program with African-American men, describe a key premise of this type of group: "Empowerment begins with a proactive assumption that people already possess the capacity to modify situations that hinder personal and interpersonal fulfillment. Rather than focussing on people's problems, empowerment emphasizes strengths and competencies" (p. 33; see also Breton, 1994b). Cox (1991) notes that "members who have survived or overcome aspects of powerlessness can inspire and motivate others" (p. 82), and as Lee (1996) asserts, "The empowerment process resides in the person, not the helper" (p. 224).

Mutual Aid

> I was scared senseless. . . . Surprisingly enough, when I was going through it, I thought I was the only one in the world. [What helped me was] a lot of sharing of information regarding what works.

A unique feature of the social work group that generates its healing qualities is the purposeful development of a democratic mutual aid system (Glassman, 1991). Through peer support, group members use experiential learning to manage feelings and to develop problem-solving strategies (Borkman, 1991; Gitterman, 1989).

> Doctors can tell you everything about the medical condition, but they can't tell you about the emotional yo-yo that you will be on for the next series of months. This group can tell you that, and

they can help you through the ups and downs. (Spousal member)

As Steinberg (2000) stated at the Toronto Symposium, "It's time to move back to social group work and discover what we already know, that mutual aid always needs to be a part of social work."

Membership

Another unique feature of social group work is the concept of membership. Lang (1979) states that the worker is a member of the group, with a role that is adaptive to the circumstances of group life. Hans Falck (1979, 1988) replaces the individual with a single person who is a member and sees social work practice in membership management terms. When membership defines relationships, self-help and mutual aid take on new depth and dimension.

Leadership and the Role of the Professional

The role of the professional in self-help, mutual aid groups is varied and controversial: "The concept of having a professional involved in a leadership role in a mutual aid group seems contradictory since this kind of group is popularly held to be professionally leaderless" (Coplon and Strull, 1983, p. 259). However, Wituk and colleagues (2000) found that only 27 percent of self-help groups were peer led with no professional involvement. Two issues, according to Coplon and Strull (1983), seem important in this discussion. The first is that groups who unite around a common medical problem tend to have more involvement with professionals. The second issue is that professionals play different roles at different stages of group development. Professionals can be helpful in setting up the group; in providing practical resources such as a meeting place, publicity, refreshments, and possible speakers; and in consulting on goals, format, and process (Coplon and Strull, 1983; Kostyk et al., 1993; Kurtz, 1990; Lurie and Shulman, 1983; Schopler and Galinsky, 1995; Wituk et al., 2000). Professional leaders can create a nonthreatening environment for communication and intervene to resolve difficulties (Wilson and Stevens, 1999), whereas "peer leaders bring their personal experience and practical problem solving skills to the group" (Kostyk et al., 1993, p. 113).

Are there drawbacks to peer leadership? Revenson and Cassel (1991) looked at the role in medical mutual help organizations and found that the demands of peer leadership may result in stress and burnout. It is here that the specialized professional leadership role in collectivity may reduce this danger: "The worker needs to identify those facets of group life or member response that are not available to the collectivity and adapt the worker role to supply the missing features" (Sulman, 1984, p. 66).

EVOLUTION OF THE PELVIC POUCH SUPPORT GROUP

First, the Staff Needed to Change . . .

Although the Pelvic Pouch Support Group had always provided a peer forum for mutual support, members tended to depend upon professional leaders to broker interactions, a pattern that had become a collective cultural norm. Professional staff needed to alter their own transactional styles to create more opportunities for members to communicate directly with one another. Staff therefore began to encourage members to interact and to respond to one another during discussions. In the networking portion of the meeting, they helped members share common experiences, trade helpful information, develop friendships, and expand their contacts for social support. These changes in the role of the professional also liberated the potential for indigenous leadership.

Emergence of Indigenous Leadership

With a shift in communication patterns, a core group of members became visible. At a network meeting, staff asked for volunteers to join a steering committee composed of peers and professionals. Several of these self-identified leaders agreed to participate, and the steering committee took ownership of a number of roles previously carried by staff alone. In response to peer members' concerns about balancing their health, work, and personal demands with leadership roles, staff reassured the members that they would share responsibilities that were burdensome. Over the course of six months, regular face-to-face meetings and e-mail discussions fostered the development of an effective task group. Short-term goals included programming, improving the meeting format, and facilitation of the support group. Peer committee members organized the program schedule for a full year in advance and advertised it in the group's newsletter that is sent to 1,500 members across Canada. They divided up the work, each taking responsibility for contacting and confirming a speaker, and for facilitating the meeting for that topic.

Changes in Meeting Format

Out of the discussion on programming came the issue of group meeting format. Because the group met infrequently, members became frustrated when participants sidelined meeting agendas by taking a lot of air time for personal issues. After exploring the problem, the committee concluded that there was too little time for networking. Thus, the group decided to shorten the presentation to allow more time for mutual aid. They also decided to delay member introductions until after the speaker. To communicate these changes and expectations to the broader network, the peer members designed a flyer that outlined the new format. In addition, they decided that the peer facilitator would take responsibility for identifying common themes during introductions and would connect those members with one another during networking time. This rotating schedule of group leadership has worked extremely well, since it gives each committee member an opportunity to experience leadership, and to develop a meaningful connection to the speaker and to the wider membership.

Enhancement of Mutual Support

The development of the steering committee subgroup has fostered mutual aid, and this in turn has precipitated changes in the patterns of communication within the collectivity as a whole. A noticeable shift is occurring within the collectivity from a psychoeducational model to a mutual aid/self-help model. In addition, spontaneous mutual support is continuing outside the group and on the inpatient ward. Members' desire to help others who are coping with the same disease has made them ambassadors for the IBD program within the hospital and in the wider community. Said one group member, "I wanted to give back—to the people who *I know* were going through what I went through."

Leadership

The transition of group leadership continues to be a work in progress. Currently, committee members participate in the buddy program and contribute ideas for the newsletter and Web site, but these aspects of the program remain the responsibility of professional staff. The steering committee has long-term goals of taking over these areas and also for developing strategies for recruitment and retention of members.

Although staff members continue to play a more active role in shaping the process than occurs in many self-help models, the role of the professional is moving from facilitator to resource person as the peer members assume responsibility for program planning and group facilitation. It is unlikely, however, that the group will completely divest itself of professional involvement because it is a community component of the IBD program designed to meet the needs of an ongoing intake of new patients and to keep members informed about new research and treatments.

CONCLUSION

In the eighteen months since its first meeting, the steering committee's motivation, commitment, and accomplishments have been impressive, especially since its peer members continue to struggle with active health problems. The efforts of staff to maximize the potential of the collectivity known as the Pelvic Pouch Support Group have taken both peer and professional members on a journey of self-discovery. The staff role has been transformed from that of group leader to group worker, and this transition has fostered communication that amplifies mutual aid and self-help. It has also decreased dependence on member-to-worker communication, and increased member-to-member interaction. More important, the mutual aid/social group work format provides a potent template for other illness support programs that employ collectivity. By enabling the empowerment and mutual aid processes in the support network, the group workers are ultimately hoping to work themselves out of a job.

REFERENCES

Borkman, T. (1991). Introduction to the special issue. *American Journal of Community Psychology, 19*(5), 643-650.

Breton, M. (1994a). On the meaning of empowerment and empowerment-oriented social work practice. *Social Work with Groups, 17*(3), 23-37.

Breton, M. (1994b). Relating competence-promotion and empowerment. *Journal of Progressive Human Services, 5*(1), 27-44.

Breton, M. (1995). The potential for social action in groups. *Social Work with Groups, 18*(2/3), 5-13.

Carlton, T. O. (1986). Group process and group work in health social work practice. *Social Work with Groups, 9*(2), 5-18.

Coplon, J. and Strull, J. (1983). Roles of the professional in mutual aid groups. *Social Casework: The Journal of Contemporary Social Work,* May, 259-266.

Cox, E. O. (1991). The critical role of social action in empowerment oriented groups. *Social Work with Groups, 14*(3/4), 77-90.

Fagan, J. and Stevenson, H. (1995). Men as teachers: A self-help program on parenting for African American men. *Social Work with Groups, 17*(4), 29-42.

Falck, H. S. (1979). The management of membership: The individual and the group. In S. L. Abels and P. Abels (Eds.), *Social Work with Groups: Proceedings of the 1979 Symposium on Social Work with Groups* (pp. 161-172). Louisville, KY: Committee for the Advancement of Social Work with Groups.

Falck, H. S. (1988). *Social Work: The Membership Perspective.* New York: Springer.

Gitterman, A. (1989). Building mutual support in groups. *Social Work with Groups, 12*(2), 5-21.

Glassman, U. (1991). The social work group and its distinct health qualities in the health care setting. *Health and Social Work, 16*(3), 203-242.

Kostyk, D., Fuchs, D., Tabisz, E., and Jacyk, W. R. (1993). Combining professional and self-help group intervention: Collaboration in co-leadership. *Social Work with Groups, 16*(3), 111-123.

Kurtz, L. F. (1990). The self-help movement: Review of the past decade of research. *Social Work with Groups, 13*(3), 101-114.

Kurtz, L. F. and Powell, T. J. (1987). Three approaches to understanding self-help groups. *Social Work with Groups, 10*(3), 69-80.

Lang, N. C. (1979). Some defining characteristics of the social work group: Unique social form. In S.L. Abels and P. Abels (Eds.), *Social Work with Groups: Proceedings of the 1979 Symposium on Social Work with Groups* (pp. 18-50). Louisville, KY: Committee for the Advancement of Social Work with Groups.

Lang, N. C. (1987). Social work practice in small social forms: Identifying collectivity. *Social Work with Groups, 9*(4), 7-32.

Lee, J. A. B. (1996). The empowerment approach to social work practice. In F. Turner (Ed.), *Social Work Treatment Interlocking Theoretical Approaches* (pp. 218-249). New York: Free Press.

Lurie, A. and Shulman, L. (1983). The professional connection with self-help groups in health care settings. *Social Work in Health Care, 8*(4), 69-76.

Parry, J. K. (1980). Group services for the chronically ill and disabled. *Social Work with Groups, 3*(1), 59-67.

Parsons, R. J. (1991). Empowerment: Purpose and practice principle in social work. *Social Work with Groups, 14*(2), 7-21.

Pernell, R. B. (1986). Empowerment and social group work. In M. Parnes (Ed.), *Innovations in Social Group Work: Feedback from Practice to Theory* (pp. 107-118). Binghamton, NY: The Haworth Press.

Revenson, T. and Cassel, B. (1991). An exploration of leadership in a medical mutual help organization. *American Journal of Community Psychology, 19*(5), 683-698.

Schopler, J. H. and Galinsky, M. J. (1995). Expanding our view of support groups as open systems. *Social Work with Groups, 18*(1), 3-10.

Steinberg, D. M. (2000). *Mutual aid and social justice.* Paper presented at the Twenty-Second Annual International Symposium on Social Work with Groups, Toronto, Canada.

Sulman, J. (1984). The worker's role in collectivity. In N. C. Lang and J. Sulman (Eds.), *Collectivity in Social Group Work* (pp. 59-67). Binghamton, NY: The Haworth Press.

Wilson, S. and Stevens, B. (1999). Introduction to groups. *Activities, Adaptation and Aging, 23*(3), 135-138.

Wituk, S., Shepherd, M. D., Slavich, S., Warren, M. L., and Meissen, G. (2000). A topography of self-help groups: An empirical analysis. *Social Work, 45*(2), 157-165.

Chapter 13

Efficacy of an Open-Ended Psychoeducational Support Group in a Health Care Setting

Sarah Ann Schuh

As a graduate social work intern, the author cofacilitated an open-ended, psychoeducational support group for caregivers of blood and marrow transplant (BMT) patients at Fairview-University Medical Center (F-UMC) in Minneapolis, Minnesota. The caregiver support group was established in February 2000 by four clinical social workers in the BMT program and serves friends and family members of patients at various stages in the transplant process.

Bone marrow transplant is a medical treatment used to treat several diseases when they have become life threatening, such as leukemias, anemias, some solid tumors, immune deficiencies, Hodgkin's disease, non-Hodgkin's lymphoma, and multiple myeloma (F-UMC, 1996; Stewart, 2000). The BMT process involves treating the patient with

> irradiation [and/or chemotherapy] to stop the production of bone marrow cells, some of which . . . [may be] diseased cells. . . . [The patient] will receive new donated stem cells from bone marrow, cord blood or peripheral blood from which new marrow cells will grow. . . . After the transplant, [the patient's] . . . new marrow should begin to produce these normal blood cells. (F-UMC, 1996, p. 4)

Many side effects and complications may occur during the bone marrow transplant process, including hair loss, mouth sores, pain, temporary mental confusion, depression, bowel and bladder problems, and infections (F-UMC, 1996; Stewart, 2000). It takes several weeks for the transplanted bone marrow to produce new cells. During these weeks, the patient's immune system is suppressed and the patient is at high risk for infection. Several precautions are taken to guard against infection: patients are in private rooms, doors to patient rooms are closed at all times, patient rooms are equipped with special air filters and positive pressure airflow to decrease the spread of germs, and thorough hand washing is required for everyone (visitors and staff) before they enter or leave patient rooms.

IMPACT OF BLOOD AND MARROW TRANSPLANTS ON PATIENTS

These patients have an illness that has become life threatening and must endure a treatment that is also life threatening. This is emphasized by Kennedy's (1993) statement that "despite advances in technology and improved morbidity and mortality rates, the psychosocial implications of this physically and emotionally arduous form of therapy are severe" (p. 104). The hospitalization stay for BMT patients varies from one week to several months (S. Dunsky, personal communication, August 24, 2001). The isolation and long hospital stay that the patients may experience in the transplant process can be a heavy psychological and emotional burden that they have never experienced prior to transplant.

The impact of the transplant experience on the patients' families is profound. "A stem cell or bone marrow transplant is a physically, emotionally, and psychologically taxing procedure for both the patient and family" (Stewart, 2000, p. 12). Patients and their families often have mixed feelings about transplant. They realize that without transplant, patient survival is limited or unlikely. Transplant offers hope, but at the same time, there are no guarantees. "The unpredictability of the course of the transplant adds to the stress, anxiety, and uncertainty they and their families experience" (Kennedy, 1993, p. 109). For these reasons, transplant is a traumatic experience physically, mentally, emotionally, and spiritually for both the patient and the family.

Caregivers of bone marrow transplant patients face many difficult issues, including being the main support for the patient; dealing with friends and family who do not understand the enormity of the situation and stress the patient and caregiver are attempting to cope with; attending to the responsibilities the patient would normally take on, such as household chores, caring for children, and monitoring the patient's medical condition; as well as adapting to the hospital culture, including the unique medical language. These issues can be overwhelming, and caregivers often need assistance in identifying areas where they need help and where to find appropriate resources.

The purpose of the caregivers' support group is to provide support to caregivers of BMT patients through education and peer support. The educational content of the group focuses on information that is vital to the caregiver role. The content provides a structural vehicle through which support and mutual aid emerge. Kennedy (1993) explained how this process unfolds: "Support groups that provide information, support, and a 'safe haven' in which to share intense feelings seem to be effective in normalizing the family's experiences, reducing their feelings of emotional isolation, and facilitating productive coping behaviors through role modeling" (p. 111).

The social worker has a crucial role in the health care setting by serving as a mediator, broker, educator, counselor, and advocate. The social worker addresses psychosocial issues with the patients and their families while providing support, education, and resources as needed. Kennedy (1993) suggests that the role of social work is essential in assisting patients and families to cope with this stress throughout the stages of treatment: pretransplant, hospitalization, and posttransplant. The social worker helps to provide continuity of care throughout the transplant process by working closely with the patients, families, and interdisciplinary staff.

LITERATURE REVIEW

In a closed support group, membership is stable. A certain number of members commit to the group and new members are not added. In contrast, in an open group there is not a membership commitment; therefore, new members are continually added while other members leave the group (Toseland and Rivas, 2001). Whether a group is open or closed affects the group purpose and the member cohesion: "In open groups, the dominant purpose is more effective coping with transitions and crises. . . . Mutuality is based more on awareness of a common condition or situation than on interpersonal relationships" (Northen, 1988, p. 138). Mutuality is the basis for mutual aid and support.

Shulman (1984) describes this mutuality as the "all-in-the-same-boat" phenomenon. It is powerful for members to hear others speak about thoughts and feelings similar to their own. This diminishes shame and normalizes their feelings so that they are "often better able to mobilize . . . [themselves] to deal with the problem productively" (Shulman, 1984, p. 166). In this way, normalization helps empower each member. Members must recognize their feelings in order to move forward into problem solving.

In closed groups, members begin to share in the leadership roles over time (Toseland and Rivas, 2001). In contrast, "there may also be rotation of workers [in an open-ended group] so that neither membership nor leadership remains stable. . . . Each session must be regarded as a group experience in itself" (Northen, 1988, p. 139). In a single-session group, the worker needs to be active in providing structural support by fostering connections among the members to facilitate support, empowerment, and mutual aid (Shulman, 1984).

Part of the social worker's role is education and supportive counseling. The patient and family receive extensive information regarding the medical aspects of the BMT treatment. Kennedy (1993) also emphasizes the necessity of "education about what to expect from a psychosocial perspective" (p. 106). Kennedy (1993, p. 106) elaborates on the purpose of this education:

> Effective education provided by the social worker about the psychosocial aspects of BMT, the hospital system, and community resources enhances the patient's and family's functioning, increases their perceived sense of control, and helps to reduce some of the anxiety that can detract from their participation in the patient's treatment.

Education helps empower patients and families to actively participate and collaborate with staff in their treatment. Several authors describe the distinct benefits of support, education, mutual aid, networking, problem solving, and empowerment in group work (Glassman, 1991; Hamlet and Read, 1990; Johnson and Stark, 1980; Kennedy, 1993; Yalom, 1995). The purpose and outcome of effective education and supportive counseling form the basis for the psychoeducational support group for caregivers of BMT patients. The open group model fits well with the inherent unpredictability of the hospital setting.

PROGRAM DESCRIPTION OF THE CAREGIVERS' SUPPORT GROUP

The four clinical social workers in the BMT department at F-UMC rotated the responsibility for facilitating the caregivers' support group, with each social worker facilitating once per month. As a social work intern, the author cofacilitated twice per month from January 2001 through April 2001. On occasion, there was a guest speaker from the interdisciplinary staff, such as a nurse, chaplain, or pharmacist, depending on the topic. When there was a speaker, the social worker continued to take an active role in facilitating discussion.

The participants in the group included family members and friends of adult and pediatric BMT patients. There were both males and females, although there were typically more females in a given group. Because caregivers included relatives and friends, the age range of participating members varied greatly from group to group. F-UMC accepts patients from across the United States as well as from around the world. There were ethnic, cultural, religious, sexual orientation, language, education, and socioeconomic variations in any given group.

Another way the membership varied was where the caregiver and patient were in the transplant process. There were caregivers of patients who were just starting the BMT process (pretransplant), those in the middle of the process (hospitalization), and those who were finishing the process (posttransplant) (Kennedy, 1993). The group composition on a given week may have included only caregivers of patients in the pretransplant stage. Other weeks the composition may have included caregivers of patients in all stages of the transplant process. In a given group, there may have been more than one caregiver present for a particular patient. For example, there were sometimes several family members in attendance at the caregivers' support group. In this manner, there were family dyads or triads represented.

An important aspect of pregroup planning was selection of topics. Topics were based on the social workers' perception of caregiver needs as well as suggestions made by caregivers. Topics have been adapted, added, or dropped based on caregiver feedback and changing needs. Topics have included caregiver concerns of anxiety, stress, and depression; how to manage nutrition, appetite, and nausea; caregiver role and changes in the family; understanding fatigue and pain management; as well as mind, body, and spirit and relaxation.

Several logistical elements of pregroup planning influenced the effectiveness of the group (see Table 13.1).

Content and format of handouts were adapted from *Home Care Guide for Cancer* (Houts, 1994). Houts (1994) presented a useful outline format to guide examination of issues in a systematic and purposeful manner. This format included the following components aimed at effective problem solving: understanding the problem, when to get professional help, what you can do to help, possible obstacles, and carrying out and adjusting your plan (Houts, 1994).

CONTENT AND PROCESS

Part of the education included discussing the significance of the advocating role of the caregiver as part of the health care team and the impact of this role on the caregiver's life. This was done through an orientation class that caregivers were invited to attend at least once. The orientation class was from 1:00 to 1:30 and the support group followed from 1:30 to 2:30. The content of the orientation included the importance of the caregiver role, preparing to be a caregiver, defining the caregiver role, discussion of types of care they would be asked to provide, the impact of the caregiver role on the caregiver, problem-solving techniques, and where to find support. These themes were carried through the support group discussion.

The educational information combined with support worked to empower and strengthen the caregivers so that they could be truly present to their loved ones. Johnson and Stark (1980) postulated that "by learning more about the disease and increasing understanding of their own feelings about it, they would theoretically become better able to accept the reality of their situation and to deal with it more directly" (p. 337).

This concept was crystallized for the author during a particular group session. Participant A stated that she had to keep being "positive" and not share any negative news because that would not help the patient get well. Participant B stated that participant A would have to

TABLE 13.1. Logistical Elements of Group Planning

Logistical Element	How This Element Affected the Group
Location	The support group was held in a conference room conveniently located next to the BMT clinic.
	The room was easily accessible.
	The location was consistent from meeting to meeting.
Time	The day and time of the meeting were consistent.
	The group started and ended on time.
Advertising	Flyers were posted each week in the BMT clinic and delivered to the inpatient rooms on brightly colored paper.
	The group meeting was automatically included in each patient's schedule of appointments during workup week.
Additional benefits	Refreshments: there was lemonade, ice water, and a variety of cookies.
	Each caregiver was given a book: *Daily Comforts for Caregivers* (Samples, 1999).
	Topical handouts were provided.
Atmosphere	The layout of the room was informal: three rectangular tables were put together to form one large rectangular table, and chairs were placed in a circle around the table.
	The size of the room was appropriate—not crowded but not so large that it seemed impersonal.
	There were paper cups, napkins, and tissues on the table.
Membership	There was no commitment necessary to participate in the group.
	A sign-in sheet was used to gauge group membership from meeting to meeting.
	Name tags were provided.

get past that and be more realistic or she would go crazy. Participant B went on to say that she had felt the same way until she realized that there would be both good days and bad days and it would be unrealistic to expect to feel and act positive all the time. The facilitator also pointed out the magical train of thought that participant A had: If she had positive thoughts, the patient would do well, and if she had negative thoughts or said negative thoughts out loud, the patient would be adversely affected. This discussion helped participant A to accept the reality of the situation and directly address her feelings of anxiety, fear, and powerlessness.

Because the group was open and both membership and leadership varied for each group session, it was necessary for the social worker to be an active facilitator. For instance, when participant A, who was in the pretransplant stage, shared a concern about the difficulty of keeping family and friends updated on the patient's condition, the social worker asked participants B and C, who were in the hospitalization and posttransplant stages, how they handled that concern. When they shared how they coped with that concern, the social worker asked participant A how it felt hearing the other participants' ideas. Participant A stated that he did not feel so bad because he was not the only one experiencing this. He also realized that he had unrealistic expectations for himself. This sharing and processing provided some relief for him. In this manner, the social worker acted to facilitate problem solving, mutual aid, and support throughout the session.

A program evaluation was developed by the BMT clinical social workers to gain feedback from participants. Although the evaluations were not distributed consistently, the feedback was used to make adjustments to the group content and format. This chapter reports findings from a preselected sample of responses from evaluations completed between February 2000 and February 2001. The responses had been collected by the author to identify what participants liked and did not like about the caregiver group. The limitation to this data is that there was not a systematic process used in collecting the findings. An attempt was made to conduct a more systematic analysis; however, the primary data had been discarded.

The majority of the program evaluations did not list anything in response to the question "What did you *not like* about the group?" Table 13.2 summarizes the themes and examples of such responses. Table 13.3 summarizes what group participants have stated they liked about the open psychoeducational support group experience.

CONCLUSION

The author recommends establishing and posting some basic ground rules, such as confidentiality, respecting others, and the right to pass

TABLE 13.2. Evaluations: Themes and Examples of What Members Did Not Like About the Group

Theme	Example
Content	Depressing to think about long-term impact of GVHD but, of course, it's better to be aware.
	Only lecture, not sharing.
Group dynamics	It is hard to have a group [member] who likes to talk, to keep [him or her] on the topic.
Meeting time and length	That it can't meet on weekends.
	Not enough time.
Membership	Wished that more people would come.
	There was a patient here for part of the time . . . [and] for whatever reason [I] was more comfortable when he left.
	Need a group with only parent caregivers of kids.

(Yalom, 1995). Group dynamics were greatly impacted when a patient was present in the caregivers' group. It was important to clearly communicate that this group was for caregivers only and that there were other opportunities for the patients to get support. The author recommends continued use of program evaluations to gather member feedback and continued teaming with interdisciplinary staff to act as guest speakers and refer caregivers to the group. Johnson and Stark (1980) found that "staff members play an essential role in making patients and families aware of the program and in encouraging them to attend" (p. 347).

The author considered this open-ended, psychoeducational support group effective based on the following indicators: attendance (there were members there each week), positive evaluations, continued support from other staff (e.g., nurses referred caregivers to the group), and witnessing the mutual aid and tremendous support the members experienced in a single session. In 1991, Glassman concluded that "group work in the health care setting has come to represent a cutting edge in group work practice" (p. 211). Ten years later, this appears still to be the case. This includes both open-ended and closed groups: "The . . . single-session group can be used in the health care setting to provide education or respond to crisis. The worker brings the crucial topic to the fore and helps everyone participate, us-

TABLE 13.3. Evaluations: Themes and Examples of What Members Did Like About the Group

Theme	Example
Atmosphere	It was very comfortable and informal. It was good to be able to ask any and all questions.
	[N]ice interaction among persons attending.
Content	Learning about the many concerns that must be confronted as a caregiver.
	One subject was covered instead of many. Very informative.
Coping	This gave me a break to talk over some of my feelings.
	Hearing how others are handling things.
Same boat	The group gave us an opportunity to realize we're not alone at all.
	Understanding/common ground [from] which to discuss.
	The easiness of talking about our situation and relating to the same things.
	Knowing that I am not alone and know[ing] that other[s] have the same problem.
	The honesty about what each person is feeling as a caregiver.
Mutual aid	Hearing out loud that it's okay for [the caregiver] . . . to take time for [himself or] herself and depend on others.
	[The] willingness of others to share thoughts and feelings.
	The opportunity to vent and receive validation and suggestions.
	The information from others going through the process.

ing directive techniques to guide the process" (Glassman, 1991, p. 204).

By providing accurate information that focused on the caregivers' needs, including a safe place to share their feelings, the support group helped people cope with the stress, trauma, and uncertainty associated with a bone marrow transplant. Feelings of isolation were diminished and a sense of mutuality developed through what Shulman (1984) referred to as the "same boat phenomenon." A sense of normalcy concerning the feelings and issues caregivers faced developed though the peer support of the group. Johnson and Stark (1980) described how normalcy develops: "[B]eing with others in similar circumstances provides a commonality of concern and a feeling of acceptance and support" (p. 337). Caregivers need accurate information concerning issues they must face, as well as emotional support, before they can move into problem solving. The caregivers' support group addresses these needs in an effective manner.

REFERENCES

Fairview-University Blood and Marrow Transplant Services (2001). *2000 Annual Report*. Minneapolis, MN: Author.

Fairview-University Medical Center (F-UMC) (1996). *Bone marrow transplant: Information for patients and families* [brochure]. Minneapolis, MN: Nursing Services.

Fairview-University Medical Center (F-UMC) (2001a). *Focus on each patient*. Retrieved from the Internet May 31, 2001: <http://www.fairviewbmt.org/focus.htm>.

Fairview-University Medical Center (F-UMC) (2001b). *A pioneer and a leader*. Retrieved from the Internet May 31, 2001: <http://www.fairviewbmt.org>.

Glassman, U. (1991). The social work group and its distinct healing qualities in the health care setting. *Health and Social Work,* 16(3), 203-212.

Hamlet, E. and Read, S. (1990). Caregiver education and support group: A hospital based group experience. *Journal of Gerontological Social Work,* 15(1/2), 75-88.

Houts, P.S. (Ed.) (1994). *Home care guide for cancer: For family and friends giving care at home*. Philadelphia, PA: American College of Physicians.

Johnson, E.M. and Stark, D.E. (1980). A group program for cancer patients and their family members in an acute care teaching hospital. *Social Work in Health Care,* 5(4), 335-349.

Kennedy, V.N. (1993). The role of social work in bone marrow transplantation. *Journal of Psychosocial Oncology,* 11(1), 103-117.

Northen, H. (1988). *Social work with groups* (Second edition). New York: Columbia University Press.

Samples, P. (1999). *Daily comforts for caregivers*. Minneapolis, MN: Fairview Press.

Shulman, L. (1984). *The skills of helping: Individuals and groups* (Second edition). Itasca, IL: F.E. Peacock Publishers, Inc.

Stewart, S.K. (2000). *Autologous stem cell transplants: A handbook for patients*. Highland Park, IL: Blood and Marrow Transplant Information Network.

Toseland, R.W. and Rivas, R.F. (2001). *An introduction to group work practice* (Fourth edition). Boston, MA: Allyn and Bacon.

Yalom, I.D. (1995). *The theory and practice of group psychotherapy* (Fourth edition). New York: Basic Books.

Index

GROWTH AND DEVELOPMENT THROUGH GROUP WORK

_____in hardbound at $29.95 (ISBN: 0-7890-2639-2)

_____in softbound at $17.95 (ISBN: 0-7890-2640-6)

Or order online and use special offer code HEC25 in the shopping cart.

COST OF BOOKS_____

☐ **BILL ME LATER;** (Bill-me option is good on US/Canada/Mexico orders only; not good to jobbers, wholesalers, or subscription agencies.)

☐ Check here if billing address is different from shipping address and attach purchase order and billing address information.

POSTAGE & HANDLING_____
(US: $4.00 for first book & $1.50 for each additional book)
(Outside US: $5.00 for first book & $2.00 for each additional book)

Signature_____

SUBTOTAL_____

☐ **PAYMENT ENCLOSED: $**_____

IN CANADA: ADD 7% GST_____

☐ **PLEASE CHARGE TO MY CREDIT CARD.**

STATE TAX_____
(NY, OH, MN, CA, IIL, N, & SD residents, add appropriate local sales tax)

☐ Visa ☐ MasterCard ☐ AmEx ☐ Discover
☐ Diner's Club ☐ Eurocard ☐ JCB

Account # _____

FINAL TOTAL_____
(If paying in Canadian funds, convert using the current exchange rate, UNESCO coupons welcome)

Exp. Date_____

Signature_____

Prices in US dollars and subject to change without notice.

NAME_____

INSTITUTION_____

ADDRESS_____

CITY_____

STATE/ZIP_____

COUNTRY_____ COUNTY (NY residents only)_____

TEL_____ FAX_____

E-MAIL_____

May we use your e-mail address for confirmations and other types of information? ☐ Yes ☐ No We appreciate receiving your e-mail address and fax number. Haworth would like to e-mail or fax special discount offers to you, as a preferred customer. **We will never share, rent, or exchange your e-mail address or fax number.** We regard such actions as an invasion of your privacy.

Order From Your Local Bookstore or Directly From
The Haworth Press, Inc.
10 Alice Street, Binghamton, New York 13904-1580 • USA
TELEPHONE: 1-800-HAWORTH (1-800-429-6784) / Outside US/Canada: (607) 722-5857
FAX: 1-800-895-0582 / Outside US/Canada: (607) 771-0012
E-mailto: orders@haworthpress.com

For orders outside US and Canada, you may wish to order through your local
sales representative, distributor, or bookseller.
For information, see http://haworthpress.com/distributors

(Discounts are available for individual orders in US and Canada only, not booksellers/distributors.)

PLEASE PHOTOCOPY THIS FORM FOR YOUR PERSONAL USE.
http://www.HaworthPress.com   BOF04